1985

W9-ABR-426

PHYSICIANS AND HOSPITALS

Physicians and Hospitals

The Great Partnership at the Crossroads
Based on the Ninth Private Sector
Conference, 1984

Edited by Duncan Yaggy and Patricia Hodgson
Foreword by William G. Anlyan

Duke University Press   Durham, 1985

Copyright © 1985 Duke University Press
All rights reserved
Printed in the United States of America
Library of Congress Cataloging in Publication Data
Private Sector Conference (9th : 1984 : Duke University Medical Center)
Physicians and hospitals.
Includes bibliographical references and index.
1. Medicine—Practice—United States—Congresses.
2. Hospitals—United States—Business management—
Congresses. 3. Hospitals—United States—Medical staff—
Congresses. I. Yaggy, Duncan. II. Hodgson, Patricia,
1942–   . III. Title. [DNLM: 1. Hospital Administration—congresses. 2. Inter-
professional Relations—
congresses. 3. Medical Staff, Hospital—congresses.
W3 PR945F 9th 1984p / WX 160 P961 1984p]
R728.P76 1984   362.1'1   84-25928
ISBN 0-8223-0639-5

Contents

Foreword

The American health care system is based on close collaboration between physicians and hospitals.

Will that partnership survive? A strong and symbiotic relationship between physicians and hospitals seems so logical and so inevitable that it is hard to imagine that it would not continue.

And yet the partnership of today is a new phenomenon. It has taken shape over the last forty years. It is the product of three developments.

One was a fresh and powerful commitment to the health of America and Americans. An early expression was the Hill-Burton Act of 1948, which built clinics and hospitals across the nation. Another was funding for the National Institutes of Health to provide organization, leadership, and support for research into the causes, treatment, and prevention of disease. With these initiatives, our society assumed for the first time a substantial and continuing responsibility for the health of its members.

Another was the health insurance movement, which was based on the premise that individuals and families should not be burdened with the increasing cost of health care services, especially inpatient services. With the rapid development of health insurance as a fringe benefit of employment, access to a full range of low-cost or no-cost services became the rule rather than the exception, and health care came to be viewed as a right rather than a privilege.

The third was the civil rights movement, which argued that access to education, employment, and other essential services and opportunities freely available to the broad majority should be extended to all citizens as a matter of right. Application of this principle to health care produced the Medicare and Medicaid programs.

These three movements interacted to produce a remarkable mandate for our physicians and hospitals: do as much as you can for as many as possible, and we will pay your costs. If you need more facilities, we will fund their construction. If you need more physicians, we will subsidize their training and the creation of an army of physician extenders to do the things that physicians are not needed to do and to reach the places where physicians are not available. Not surprisingly, the number of patients served and the volume of services provided grew rapidly.

Physicians and hospitals worked together as never before. Physicians became more and more dependent on hospitals, both for increasingly sophisticated services and facilities and for the opportunity to earn substantial incomes efficiently. Hospitals relied increasingly on physicians, both for the patients essential to their growth and financial health and for the management of high technology ancillary services.

As the costs mounted and the evidence of excesses accumulated, checks on the supply of services and facilities were introduced, the practice patterns of physicians were monitored, and the mandate was qualified: "Do all you can" became "Do as much as is necessary and cost beneficial." But the thrust and the effect remained the same. Access to a widening range of health care services was extended to an increasing share of a growing population, and the costs continued to climb.

Strains in the relationship have appeared only in the last few years. They are the consequence of several forces, including:

—medical advances that allow outpatient delivery of services previously provided on an inpatient basis, as well as shorter lengths of stay for those admitted.

—a steady increase in the supply of practicing physicians. In North Carolina, for example, the supply continues to grow five times faster than the state's population.

—reimbursement limits that compel hospitals to monitor, and adjust where possible, the practice patterns of their physicians.

—efforts by third-party payers to reduce hospital utilization. These initiatives, which include prior authorization for admissions, outpatient testing, review of weekend utilization, and prepaid plans, enlist physicians in the effort to eliminate unnecessary admissions, to postpone necessary admissions until active treatment is to begin, and to reduce the length of stay.

The signs of strain are already visible: physicians organize free-standing ambulatory care facilities to compete with the service of their own hospitals; hospitals testify against certificate of need applications filed by their physicians; hospitals organize satellite clinics to assure a flow of patients; etc.

The forces generating these strains are growing steadily stronger, and they seem certain to exercise a powerful influence in the years to come. The Ninth Private Sector Conference met to examine the relations between physicians and hospitals, to ask whether the collaboration that has developed over the last forty years will continue, give way to competition, or take new forms. We also wanted to consider the implications for our health care system, for those it serves, and for society.

As you will see, the discussion was far-reaching and provocative.

Without the support of the Duke Endowment, which has sponsored the Private Sector Conferences since their inception in 1977, this book would not have been possible.

William G. Anlyan, M.D.

Participants

John E. Affeldt, M.D., President, Joint Commission on Accreditation of Hospitals

William G. Anlyan, M.D., Chancellor for Health Affairs, Duke University

Joseph F. Boyle, M.D., President-elect, American Medical Association

Michael Bromberg, Executive Director, Federation of American Hospitals

John W. Colloton, Director and Assistant to the President for Statewide Health Services, University of Iowa Hospitals and Clinics

John A. D. Cooper, M.D., President, Association of American Medical Colleges

Patricia Danzon, Associate Professor, Center for Health Policy Research and Education and Institute for Policy Sciences, Duke University

Edgar Davis, Vice-President, Corporate Affairs Division, Eli Lilly and Company

James M. Denny, Chairman of the Board, Pearle Health Services, Inc.

Merlin K. DuVal, M.D., President, Associated Health Systems

C. Douglas Eavenson, Assistant Director, Employee Benefits and Services, General Motors Corporation

Paul M. Ellwood, Jr., M.D., President, InterStudy

Alain Enthoven, Mariner S. Eccles Professor of Public and Private Management, Graduate School of Business, Stanford University

E. Harvey Estes, Jr., M.D., Chairman, Department of Community and Family Medicine, Duke University Medical Center

ASHLEY H. GALE, JR., Director, Hospital and Child Care Sections, The Duke Endowment

ELI GINZBERG, Ph.D., Director, Conservation of Human Resources, Columbia University

C. ROLLINS HANLON, M.D., Director, American College of Surgeons

CLARK HAVIGHURST, Professor, School of Law, Duke University

DAVID KINZER, President, Massachusetts Hospital Association

JOSEPH LIPSCOMB, JR., Ph.D., Associate Professor of Public Policy Studies and Community and Family Medicine, Duke University

DONALD MACNAUGHTON, President, Hospital Corporation of America

BILLY G. MCCALL, Deputy Executive Director and Secretary, The Duke Endowment

J. ALEXANDER MCMAHON, President, American Hospital Association

WALTER J. MCNERNEY, Professor of Health Policy, Kellogg Graduate School of Management, Northwestern University

ALAN NELSON, M.D., Trustee, American Medical Association

STANLEY NELSON, President, Henry Ford Health Care Corporation

DAVID J. OTTENSMEYER, M.D., President, Lovelace Medical Foundation

UWE E. REINHARDT, Ph.D., Woodrow Wilson School of Public and International Affairs, Princeton University

B. L. RHODES, Executive Vice-President, Kaiser Foundation Health Plan, Inc.

DAVID E. ROGERS, M.D., President, The Robert Wood Johnson Foundation

PAUL G. ROGERS, Esq., Hogan & Hartson Law Firm

JAMES H. SAMMONS, M.D., Executive Vice-President, American Medical Association

JACK K. SHELTON, Manager, Employee Insurance Department, Ford Motor Company

ROSEMARY A. STEVENS, Department of History and Sociology of Science, University of Pennsylvania

JOHN D. THOMPSON, Department of Epidemiology and Public Health, Yale University

ANDREW G. WALLACE, M.D., Vice-Chancellor for Health Affairs, Duke University

RICHARD S. WILBUR, M.D., Executive Vice-President, Council of Medical Specialty Societies
DAVID G. WILLIAMSON, Executive Vice-President of Development, Hospital Corporation of America
JOHN IGLEHART, Rapporteur

The Cybernetics of Our System

ANDREW G. WALLACE, M.D.

It seems reasonable to assume that our topic for this conference, "Physicians and Hospitals: The Great Partnership at a Cross-roads," would not have been chosen if it was not perceived as a problem. I am new to the ranks of medical administrators, while there are others at this conference who have been in the trenches longer and viewed our subject from a wider range of experiences. Some have actually developed strategies to relieve the stress that is implied by our title. For these reasons I have chosen to search my own background for experiences that might complement yours and provide each of us with a useful framework for thinking about our topic. There is a risk in this departure, but there is also a compelling need to orient our dialogue toward causes rather than symptoms, toward a process that seeks solutions as opposed to palliative procedures.

Consider that the interface between doctors and hospitals is just one special case of a much broader issue: how to understand and constructively steer the behavior of complex systems. As in any system made up of interdependent parts, the interaction of the components of the system will determine how we progress from the present to the future. Most systems that I am familiar with are characterized by change, growth, and goal seeking and are governed by feedback. For example, feedback is a characteristic of the operation of biological systems, of interpersonal relations, of corporate behavior, and of large social systems. I believe that there are lessons we can learn from those who have studied feedback, and that these lessons have application to the problem we are discussing and to the formulation of policies that will lead to real solutions.

My first exposure to the concept of feedback came in the study of biological systems. As a student in biochemistry, I struggled to memorize a host of biosynthetic pathways responsible for generating compounds essential to the function of living cells. I have forgotten many of the specifics, but I remember the important concepts, including that of end product inhibition. The principle is illustrated by figure 1.1. In this example the conversion of substrate A to intermediary B is catalyzed by enzyme E_1, and the conversion of intermediary B to the final product C is catalyzed by enzyme E_2. The important point is that the level of product C modifies the activity of enzyme E_1. This intrinsically simple control mechanism recurs throughout biological systems and is, in fact, the basic process by which physiologic systems achieve equilibrium.

Claude Bernard, who is regarded by many as the father of modern physiological thought, wrote the following in the middle of the nineteenth century:

> Science should always explain obscurity and complexity by clearer simple ideas. . . . There is an arrangement in the living being, a kind of regulated activity which must never be neglected, . . . it is in truth the most striking characteristic of living beings. . . . It is as if there existed a pre-established design . . . such that though considered separately each physiological process is dependent upon the general forces of nature . . . yet taken in relation to other processes it reveals a special bond and seems directed by some invisible guide. . . .

The "invisible guide" in Bernard's work and thought became the basis for the concept of feedback control in biology. Does this concept apply to the arena in which doctors and hospitals work? I think it does. Physicians are products of an educational system

1. End product inhibition.

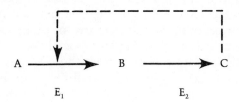

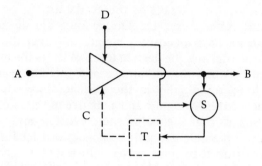

2. Model delay in a feedback loop.

that catalyzes the conversion of students into medical manpower. Yet today it is primarily physicians, from both practice and academia, who are calling for a reduction in the rate of production of their own kind. Hospitals, too, are the product of forces that over the last twenty-five to fifty years have called for expansion of facilities and greater access. Yet today, either in the open or by subtle means, hospitals are exerting pressure to constrain their own further proliferation. The dynamic of feedback is with us.

For a period of time science was satisfied to look for evidence of feedback, or its lack, in various biological events. But soon the process of feedback itself became the subject of intense investigation. There are concepts derived from this effort to understand the regulation of biological systems that have their analogies in social systems. We have learned that feedback is often triggered not by the level of a product per se, but rather by the difference between the actual output of a reaction and either the genetically determined or evolutionarily desired level of output. We have learned that the compensating force in a feedback loop is related to this difference but not necessarily equal or directly proportional to it. We have learned that the change in the level of product over time, when a process is perturbed, is influenced importantly by the delay in the feedback loop (figure 1.2). In this figure A is the level of substrate. B is the level of product. S is a sensor designed to detect the difference between B and its desired level D. The compensatory force C is related to this difference, but delayed in time and quantifiably related to the difference by a transfer function or process T.

Consider for a moment that this model might describe either the production of physicians or the availability or cost of some arbitrary unit of health service. Do we know the desired level of product? Do we have a sensor adequate to detect the difference between the actual and the desired level? What is the quantitative relationship between this difference and the compensatory signal? How long is the delay in the feedback loop—for example between the GMENAC report and a change in the rate of production of physicians that is equal to their attrition rate?

The range of possible dynamic responses of a feedback system when you perturb it in some way is illustrated in figure 1.3. We see that (1) shows what would happen without feedback, (2) is the desired response of a stable system with appropriate feedback, and (3) is a system with appropriate compensation but long delay in the feedback line. Which curve best describes the growth of physicians or of medical costs?

The word "cybernetics" is newer than the concept of feedback. Norbert Wiener, a mathematician from M.I.T., began to work on the theory of messages about forty years ago. He was interested in engineering, in language, in biology, and in psychology. He created the word *cybernetics*, which was derived from the Greek "Kubernetes," meaning "to steer." In 1950 he wrote a book, *The Human Use of Human Beings*,[1] in which he developed the theses that social systems could be understood only through a study of feedback messages; that stability required that the results of one's

[1]   Norbert Wiener, *The Human Use of Human Beings* (Garden City, N.Y.: Doubleday, 1954).

3. Possible dynamic response of a feedback system.

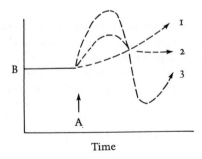

Time

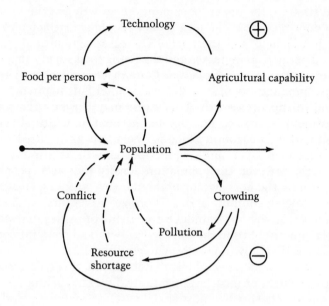

4. Forces that change social systems from a growth mode to an equilibrium mode.

actions be communicated back as a part of the information upon which we continue to act; that cybernetics is the only force that prevents the natural tendency toward disorganization.

Jay Forrester, who is also at M.I.T., applies cybernetics to social systems. About twelve years ago he wrote *World Dynamics*,[2] a book based on studies sponsored by the Club of Rome and best known because of its doomsday predictions. Forrester is a member of a community of model builders—global models designed to capture and understand and forecast the behavior of complex social systems such as a corporation, a city, the economy, or the world. His thesis is that social systems belong to a class of multilooped feedback systems and that it is possible to construct in the laboratory realistic models that describe and predict their behavior.

Although simplified by excluding a multiplicity of factors that actually operate in complex social systems, figure 1.4 illustrates the nature of forces that ultimately change such systems from a

[2]   Jay Forrester, *World Dynamics* (Cambridge, Mass.: Wright-Allen Press, 1971).

growth mode to an equilibrium mode through feedback.[3] In the illustration, the upper loops promote growth and the lower loops produce restraint. The idea is that people are attracted to an area of fertile land and their labor increases agricultural capability. Food per person increases and the rising food supply supports further increases in population. Growth continues until the marginal productivity of an additional worker fails to produce enough food to support growth. This stress may trigger a temporary investment in new technology to augment agricultural capability, and with this capability food per person is again lifted above the subsistence level and population growth continues. During growth, however, the population density increases, people begin to occupy the best agricultural land, and crowding creates pollution, social conflict, and a shortage of resources. The consequence of growth is to induce ever-rising pressures to restrain further growth. In time the forces of growth and restraint come into balance, and growth gives way to equilibrium.

Forrester's thesis would be that models of this type describe the growth curve of most organizations. By extrapolation, his model also predicts that for most social systems including world population there is a limit to growth. My reason for elaborating the Forrester philosophy is my belief that it has application to the health care enterprise and to the issue we are here to discuss— physicians and hospitals. Whether you view health care as a system unto itself or as a part of a larger social system, several generalizations can be drawn from the dynamic behavior of complex systems.

1. Together we have cultivated an expectation that our enterprise can promote health, increase longevity, and increase productivity. The accomplishments of the past give credence to that argument. We are now investing in technology as an expression of the continuing expectation of what can be accomplished through the health enterprise. The public has supported that view and so we are operating in the upper area of this particular growth curve, an area of positive feedback and growth. On the other hand, any thoughtful projection of what changes our enterprise is likely to produce in terms of health, longevity or productivity over the next fifty years compared with the last fifty years indicates that

[3] Jay Forrester, "Churches at the Transition Between Growth and World Equilibrium," *Zygon; Journal of Religion and Science* 7(1972):145. Reprinted with permission of the author and publisher.

those changes are going to be smaller, more difficult to accomplish, and more costly.

In addition, we are bumping into a progressive series of ethical questions. We have technology today that we know how to use but not when to use. Nowhere is that dilemma greater in the operation of the hospital than at the two ends of the age spectrum.

My point is that we're beginning to see some of the forces of negative feedback. We're beginning to see some of the forces of restraints on our system and, from my perspective, the growth curve of the health care enterprise is beginning to turn to a slower rate of growth.

2. Forrester points out that the transition from growth to equilibrium is always characterized by stress. One reason is that problems previously solved by expansion now must be solved by setting priorities within the constraint of relatively fixed resources. Policies that served well during growth no longer apply. I suggest that the stress today between physicians and hospitals is a predictable symptom of a system in transition from growth to equilibrium. If that hypothesis is correct, let us not assume that the supply of new physicians, new entrepreneurial practice styles, and new hospital strategies will all be additive. There will be winners and losers, survivors and casualties in the new medicine.

3. A third concept that can be drawn from the Forrester view is the "counter-intuitive behavior of social systems." The basic idea is that in the absence of a conceptual model that describes and quantifies the relation between all components of a system, people of good intentions will establish and follow policies designed to optimize the performance of their own component believing that in so doing they will help to improve the operation of the entire system. When a system is in trouble and these operative policies are identified, combined, and allowed to interact, the consequences usually mimic the actual difficulty of the system.[4]

One of my fears is that as doctors, hospitals, government, and business seek new ways to optimize their own conditions, in the absence of an adequate understanding of the negative consequences of their actions for other components in the system, the health care system as a whole becomes vulnerable to a worsening condition. The capacity of doctors to optimize their practice style without regard to hospital operating costs is legend, and the ca-

[4] Jay Forrester, "Counterintuitive Behavior of Social Systems," *Technology Review* 73(1971):52–68.

pacity of hospitals to adopt strategies to cut costs without appreciating the adverse impact on doctors is also legend. What we seem to lack is a model that defines these relationships, that allows us to predict the short-term and long-term consequences of a particular action and to seek policies that may require compromise of individual goals in the short run for the sake of overall system performance in the longer run.

I will conclude this brief and risky venture into the world of cybernetics with a few thoughts.

1. The principle of feedback is fundamental to understanding the behavior of simple and complex systems. It applies to the interface between physicians and hospitals and to the interface between health care and other components of our social system. It is our responsibility to explore relationships that cultivate common objectives, promote feedback, achieve synergy, and avoid adversarial postures.

2. If doctors and hospitals are interdependent, then the basic question is whether or not they are coupled by policies that facilitate feedback and optimal achievement of a shared goal. I believe the linkage leaves much to be desired, and the perception that our goals differ contributes significantly to the stress between doctors and hospitals.

3. Even if the feedback loops exist, there is reason to ask whether the phase lag between a particular action and its consequences isn't so long that the feedback is ineffective. The best example I can think of is, how long will it take to bring the rate of production of physicians into balance with the rate of attrition?

4. I confess I do not know what the relationship between the vast range of physician practice styles that is emerging and the equally vast range of hospital styles should be. My current view is that the plethora of styles is more a symptom of stress than a solution. They smack of encircled wagons, or self-optimization without a clear vision of their effect on other parts or on total system functions. I admit that some surgery can be done well and at less unit cost in a surgicenter, but I haven't been convinced that total health costs of a community will be lowered. A "doc-in-a-box" may do well today, but what will the quality of his practice be ten years from now, how will he know, and what will we do?

5. I return to Forrester's model because I believe we are, or shortly will be, headed for an excess health care capacity relative to resources, a host of negative feedback forces designed to reduce the rate of growth, and predictably a period of increasing stress.

We seem to lack a conceptual model of the whole health care system, one that allows us to predict the distant consequences of a given policy. We simply have not yet faced the reality that to simultaneously seek quality, equity of distribution, freedom for providers, and cost control is impossible. A group such as this one gathered here has the clout to recommend policies that will constrain growth and the proliferation of dysynergy within the health care system. A group such as this has the capacity to create a model that defines the relation between components of our system and to estimate the consequences of a given policy on other components and on the performance of the total system. A conference such as this should set for itself the goal of understanding the relation between doctors and hospitals and formulating strategies that will facilitate their interaction toward the broader social purpose both serve. Physicians and hospitals are interdependent, and they are mutually dependent on achieving that broader purpose.

2

The Uneasy Alliance

JOHN D. THOMPSON

I begin with a hypothesis: a hospital is a medical-social institution, and the primary function of the trustees is to mediate across the hyphen. They attempt to do this while preserving the financial viability of their institution and maintaining the quality of care given by a variety of professionals.

The types of pressures from each of the two groups, i.e., from society and from the medical professional, particularly the hospital staff, have changed radically over the 120-year existence of the modern hospital. Early hospitals in the United States, not surprisingly, adopted the nonreligious models of ownership and organization emerging in England. The nonprofit form quite similar to that found in, among others, Guy's Hospital and St. Thomas' Hospital in London became the dominant form of ownership and governance. The boards of governors that ran the two hospitals in England set the pattern for the development of the early hospitals both in England and in the United States. Guy's Hospital was founded by a merchant, and it was this class that founded the Massachusetts[1] and Pennsylvania[2] general hospitals in this country. Let there be no confusion: St. Thomas' began as one of the five royal hospitals, but the king did very little to support, maintain, or manage it; he merely granted the charter to petitioning citizens of London. Hospitals in the early days were considered "venerable charities," and of the five royal hospitals only two were for the general care of the sick poor. Of the other three, one was for the care and schooling of orphans; one was dedicated to

[1] Fred A. Washburn, *The Massachusetts General Hospital* (Boston: Houghton Mifflin, 1939).
[2] Francis R. Packard, *Some Account of the Pennsylvania Hospital* (Philadelphia: Engle Press, 1938).

the care of prisoners, and the other was for the treatment of the insane. Later, during the reign of Charles II, a sixth hospital was chartered for the care of pensioners of the armed forces.

The medical staff of these hospitals, by and large, were considered a special class of part-time employees. They were, in most instances, paid a salary. When the governors felt they were not earning that salary, it was not unusual for them, as at St. Thomas' in 1858, to lay down conditions of performance. The board of governors specified that surgeons should reside within one mile of the hospital during their "taking in weeks," that patients should be admitted every day instead of once a week, and that physicians and surgeons should visit the wards at 8:30 or 9:00 a.m.[3] In Guy's Hospital, two physicians were dismissed because they disagreed with the governors' decision to start a Nightingale-type nursing school at the hospital.[4] During this period, then, one could say that the social role of the hospital was predominant and that the "power" of the physicians outside of treating their patients was rather limited. This was true in spite of the fact that both St. Thomas' and Guy's had medical schools.

To represent the physicians and surgeons, so-called "medical committees" were formed in some of the hospitals in England. These precursors of medical staff organizations began to carve out those areas of concern in medical practice and represented in a more focused manner the interests of the physicians and surgeons, particularly with regard to teaching and research.

The situation in England in 1860, according to Brian Abel-Smith, was that "the general hospitals had developed a system of bipartite administration. Power was divided between a 'house committee' (board of governors) and a 'medical committee' (medical staff). Each had authority for independent action within a limited sphere, but if it came to a clash of interests, the house committee had the last word. This administrative structure represented the uneasy alliance upon which the voluntary system was based."[5]

There were major differences between the early hospitals in the United States and their precursors in Great Britain. The distances

[3] F. G. Parsons, *The History of St. Thomas's Hospital*, vol. 3 (London: Methuen, 1936), p. 140.
[4] Hujohn A. Ripman, ed., *Guy's Hospital* (London, 1951).
[5] Brian, Abel-Smith, *The Hospitals 1800–1948* (London: Heinemann, 1964), p. 224.

of social class between the governors and the medical staff did not define the relationships between the two bodies in America anywhere nearly as strongly as in England. Early problems in the United States were concerned with the foundation of the hospitals, and physicians were much involved in this process;[6] management of hospitals, once founded, was often entrusted to outstanding physicians. Further, with the exception of the director, physicians were not paid by the hospital, and it was not until some time later that they were allowed to charge professional fees to their patients.[7] The uneasy alliance, indeed, came to characterize governance of the hospitals in the United States, but at a later date.

The modern hospital was born in the decade between 1860 and 1870. In June 1860, the first class of probationers arrived at St. Thomas' School of Nursing, founded by Florence Nightingale and financed by the Nightingale Fund. In 1867 Joseph Lister published in *Lancet* the results of his work in Scotland on the antiseptic treatment of amputations. Though it was to be some time before the full implications of the latter changes were to be felt, evidence of them can be drawn from a biography of Dr. Lister:

> Lister came to London in 1877, and at that time the majority of patients preferred to undergo operations in their own homes, an arrangement which favored the general practitioner who then retained the case under his own control. It was essential to the success of Lister's method, however, that each dressing should be conducted under the same rigid precautions as the operation, and by accommodating his patients near him, he was able to give them the close attendance which the technique demanded.[8]

Dr. Lister found it necessary to open a "nursing home" or private hospital to treat such patients.

There are three implications in this simple paragraph. First, the well-to-do patients had to be hospitalized as well as the sick poor.

[6]   J. D. Thompson and G. Goldin, *The Hospital: A Social and Architectural History* (New Haven: Yale University Press, 1975).
[7]   Henry C. Burdett, *Pay Hospitals and Paying Wards throughout the World* (Philadelphia: P. Blakiston, 1880).
[8]   D. Guthrie, *Lord Lister, His Life and Doctrine* (Edinburgh: Livingstone, 1949), p. 92.

They could no longer be treated in their homes. Second, rigorous postoperative care by surgeons was essential to the well-being of their patients. No longer could they turn them over to the dressers or general practitioners once the operation was finished. Third, the surgeon, who could now operate safely, became the leading power in the hospital itself. This was particularly true following the discovery of asepsis by Von Bergman.[9] In 1884 a large private hospital was built at Kiel "expressly for the purpose of carrying out this technique. Dr. Gustav Niebuhr separated the operating theaters as being 'dirty' and 'clean' while the air of the theaters was sterilized by heat and by passing it through cotton filters."[10] This first major technological revolution eventually resulted in pressures upon the boards of trustees in U.S. hospitals to provide the proper facilities, equipment, and staff for surgeons to carry out their newly established treatment regimens.

Almost as important, the gradual acceptance by, and exclusive ownership of, the germ theory by the medical world gave that profession a provable theory at the core of its science and enhanced the profession's credibility to society in general. It legitimized the takeover of preventive medicine and public health from the engineers and social reformers who had promoted the sanitary revolution. Although of limited use in therapy, except for the surgeons, the germ theory changed the way the profession viewed itself and set a professional strategy of diagnosis and prevention of the major causes of death for the next decades.

In the hospital the era of the surgeon radically altered the balance of power between the trustees and the medical staff. This was particularly true in the United States where, unlike in England, no formal differentiation between the two branches of medicine existed. The first task, therefore, was to distinguish the surgeons from the rest of the medical profession. This task was undertaken by the American College of Surgeons. The problem was that hospital records were so "meager and poor that most applicants for fellowship in the college could not produce satisfactory reports of the 50 major and 50 minor operations required for fellowship."[11] Medical records had to become standardized through an organization of the medical staff that allowed the staff

[9]   George Rosen, *A History of Public Health* (New York: MD Publications, 1958).
[10] Guthrie, *Lord Lister*, p. 102.
[11] Malcolm T. MacEachern, *Hospital Administration* (Berwyn, Ill.: Physician Record Co., 1962), p. 1175.

to identify those who were operating and set standards for the quality of surgical care given in the hospital itself.

It was in this early stage of development that Codman advanced a shared quality control system with the suggestion that "each prominent hospital . . . appoint an efficiency committee consisting of a trustee, a member of the (medical) staff and a superintendent."[12] This committee was really what we would call now an "effectiveness" committee, since its main charge was to investigate the end result of hospital care through follow-up studies of the condition of the patient one year after hospitalization. Instead, a formalized structure was established that, though it had in the main positive effects on hospital care, placed the responsibility of monitoring care exclusively with the medical staff. This separate structure was strengthened with every subsequent advance in medical science, particularly when the nonsurgical specialties finally achieved a major therapeutic breakthrough with the discovery of antibiotics,[13] starting with the application of the sulfa drugs in the late thirties. Such a structure was not only compatible with the emerging pattern of broad subspecialization in medicine, but was legitimized when the Joint Commission on Hospital Accreditation was founded, strengthening the economic base for specialists within the hospital. The selection of one individual according to a set of criteria, however, automatically entails the exclusion of others. This process requires a strong, well-written set of medical staff bylaws if these practices are to be defensible in the courts.

The growth of this separate medical structure in U.S. hospitals and the economic interdependence of the two bodies tilted the relationship between society and medicine as illustrated in Paul Starr's recent book.[14] What was its effect on the "mediator"—the boards of trustees? To return to Abel-Smith's paradigm, it became more difficult for the "house committees" to exercise their final authority in the light of redefined areas "for independent action." The critical factor became the precise definition of the "limited spheres" of authority and responsibility.

An enormous amount of rhetoric was devoted to describing the relationship between the trustees and the medical staffs, particu-

---

[12]   E. A. Codman, *The Shoulder* (Boston, 1934), p. xviii.
[13]   Lewis Thomas, *The Youngest Science* (New York: Viking, 1983), pp. 3–5.
[14]   Paul Starr, *The Social Transformation of American Medicine* (New York: Basic Books, 1982).

larly the organization of the latter. Descriptive terms were used, such as "self government,"[15] and "freedom of action,"[16] under by-laws either separate from or part of those of the hospital that should be like a "well fitting girdle, strong enough for support but loose enough to permit reasonable movement,"[17] and headed by a chief of staff as a liaison person with the administration and the board.[18] Even the form of organization that attempts to remove the "gauze curtain" between the trustees and the medical staff by requiring that the chief of staff be appointed by and responsible to the board didn't really become widely accepted in U.S. hospitals. Goldwater's joint conference committee[19] didn't clarify the relationship much either.

To a modern manager concerned with diagramming authority and responsibility, the notion of an autonomous medical staff dealing with administration through a joint conference committee (not joint management or administrative committee) was an anathema. It appeared more like two independent nations negotiating than one bipartite organization dealing in patient care. How could the trustees mediate between the demands of society and medicine if they could not manage their own institutions?

In the midst of all this confusion of authority and responsibility, two clear characteristics of the hospital's organization appear throughout its history. The strengthened role of the medical staff flew under the banner of quality of care, and the staff members were presumed to be ignorant of financial matters in the hospital. The penannt for the board of trustees was that of public trust for the resources committed to them by society. Board members were presumed to know as little about the quality of medical care as the staff members were presumed to know of financial matters— "it is unreasonable to expect visiting physicians and surgeons to devote time to a study of the details of hospital expenditures, a study foreign to their daily thought,"[20] said Goldwater in an earlier day. Both sides were to be sheltered from the concerns of the other. The *Darling* decision clearly closed the era of nonconcern

[15] Report on Physicians-Hospital Relations, June 1964. Council on Medical Service, Committee on Medical Facilities of the American Medical Association, Chicago, 1964, as quoted in C. W. Eisele, ed., *The Medical Staff in the Modern Hospital* (New York: McGraw-Hill, 1967), p. 3.

[16] Ibid., p. 4.

[17] Ibid., p. 17.

[18] Ibid., p. 37.

[19] S. S. Goldwater, *On Hospitals* (New York: Macmillan, 1949), p. 93.

[20] Ibid., p. 91.

of the board for quality of care. What is going to change the attitude of the staff toward the financial implications of medical practice?

How did society view this growth and change? Did it feel as though its concerns were being mediated by the hospitals' boards? Though it is difficult to answer these questions, many who spoke for "society" presented their own points of view, whether they reflected general societal concerns or not. The various levels of government are not only legitimate spokesmen for society but can act in society's interest. The federal government in its various perceptions about hospitals in the United States passed from almost unqualified approval to punitive restrictions from the immediate postwar period to the present date. Though there was some concern that higher quality of hospital care could be achieved through a more regionalized system and that a more equal distribution of hospitals could achieve greater equity of access and a better distribution of physicians, the federal government firmly placed its trust in voluntary hospital boards with the passage of the Hill-Burton program of governmental construction grants. After the passage of Medicare and Medicaid in 1966, however, that trust began to erode visibly each year as the costs of Medicare began to spiral. In desperation, permanent programs were mounted to control the *supply* of hospital facilities in P.L. 93-641 and to influence *demand* for care through the PSRO legislation. These laws reflected the perception that trustees and physicians were acting in concert to drive up the costs of hospital care without any perceptible increase in the quality of that care. The famous phrase in P.L. 93-641 that its goal was to achieve the highest quality of hospital care for the lowest possible cost was a clear sign to the hospitals of the inseparability of the concerns of the trustees and medical staff. In addition to the federal attack on rising costs, several states passed different forms of hospital cost control, with or without the assistance of federal funds.

What about society itself? What were its perceptions at this time? Fortunately we have two fairly recent public surveys, one from 1978[21] and the other from 1983,[22] both from Louis Harris and Associates. Both deal with various aspects of health care, the

[21]   Louis Harris and Associates for Hospital Affiliates International, *Hospital Care in America*, April 1978.
[22]   Louis Harris and Associates for the Equitable Life Assurance Society of the United States, *The Equitable Healthcare Survey*, August 1983.

first concentrating on hospitals and the second on more general aspects of health care.

The first study was carried out at the time the Carter Administration was recommending its cost control legislation. The survey revealed the public opposed additional federal regulation of hospitals in spite of a deep dissatisfaction with doctors' fees and hospital charges that were perceived as very high. On the other hand, the public's perception of quality of health care was most favorable: 78 percent of the sample reported being very or somewhat satisfied with the quality of health care given to patients staying in hospitals. Further, the quality of care in church-related and other voluntary hospitals was higher than in government hospitals or those owned by professional management companies.

The more recent survey also probed public satisfaction with the quality and cost of health care. Public perceptions of the quality of health care continued positive: 77 percent of the public was either very satisfied or somewhat satisfied in 1983. On the other hand, hospital costs seemed increasingly unreasonable:[23] in 1978, 50 percent of the public sample rated hospital costs as either "somewhat unreasonable" or "very unreasonable"; by 1983, these judgments had risen to 63 percent, the largest increase being in the "very unreasonable" category from 25 percent to 36 percent.

The board's effectiveness has been mixed. While successfully negotiating professional standards in line with society's expectations for quality of care, the board has failed to respond to society's concern for the costs of the care given in its institution. Furthermore, its own bipartite management structure has prevented the board from understanding the relationship between cost and quality, or even from admitting that there is one. The fear that any decrease in costs is necessarily linked to decreases in quality paralyzes such an inquiry. This is in spite of the fact that within their own hospital there is evidence of large variations in the cost of treating patients with the same medical conditions without any effect on the end results of that treatment.

The "gauze curtain" between the medical records room and the financial office must disappear, allowing both the trustees and the physicians to relate the costs of treatment to the quality of care. Armed with this information, both parties to the uneasy alliance will be managing patient care with a common set of

[23]   Ibid., p. 22.

professional and fiscal standards. That is the true meaning of case management. In this fashion, the hospitals can progress from how they got where they are to where they should be, responding to the perceptions of society and the demands of medical science.

Response

ROSEMARY A. STEVENS

I'm not at all sure that doctors and hospitals have been great partners in the past, and I'm not sure that we are at the crossroads either. But one of the uses of history is to help us understand the present and gear up for the future, so I'm not going to quibble about the title of our conference. I would like to make some points about the dichotomies that we tend to perceive between doctors and hospitals and, in Dr. Thompson's paper, between physicians and boards of trustees.

I'd like to make points in three areas that have played a part in how we got to where we are. These three areas are separation of hospitals and medical financing, a very artificial separation; the growing technique of hospital management, which I think raises a whole host of compelling questions; and changes in the broader environment.

The separation of hospitals and medical financing has been a fascinating phenomenon in American medicine. Perhaps the real point to be raised in the history of the relationship between hospitals and physicians is the dependence of American hospitals on paying patients—almost from the beginning of the period that Dr. Thompson described. Most American hospitals were never charities. They were founded from the beginning to serve paying patients. Most American hospitals have very little endowment. They have always thought of themselves as businesses.

Boards of trustees historically have had very little to do with trusteeship. Throughout their history they have had trouble defining their role, which is now becoming much more explicit in terms of its managerial aspects.

As far as the technique of hospital management is concerned, I don't see a simple dichotomy here. I see the administrator becoming very important as a mediating factor in the thirties, rising in importance in the forties, and becoming an expert with the expertise required for the reimbursement systems of the sixties, seventies, and eighties. Administration is now becoming a third force with a separate set of skills rivaling medical skills in power, if not in importance.

A third set of issues relates to the broader environment. First, there is the recent development of hospital systems that are alternative kinds of hospital care. They provide great and new roles for physicians as employees, as entrepreneurs, and as committee members. Second, there is the impact of the relatively large physician supply. Third, I see schisms arising within the medical profession that are going to affect the relationships between physicians and hospitals: variations in practices within medical specialties and conflicts of view between older physicians and younger physicians, between poorer physicians and richer physicians, and between those who are entrenched in hospital staffs and those who have difficulty getting places. I worry that we may be creating a generation of debt-ridden cynics coming out of medical school with impossible expectations; they, too, will affect attitudes in the future.

Finally, I think we're going to see changes in the nature of decision making. We're going to see within medicine the need to consult many different groups—not only physicians, administrators, and boards of trustees, but nurses, businesses, other health professions, and other licensed independent practitioners. Already we see conflict; not conflict between good guys and bad guys or rational people and irrational people, but conflicts between rational points of view expressed by different groups and different individuals. Decision making in and outside hospitals is inevitably a constant renegotiation of goals, a constant renegotiation of procedures, a constant effort to define what we mean by value in medical care. Where are physicians and hospitals going to be in all of this?

I'm not really very happy with the idea either of an uneasy alliance or of a simple partnership. Rather, I think we are entering an era of constantly shifting alliances and constantly shifting partnerships, a pattern I think we're going to be living with at least through the end of the century.

The question remains, What role will physicians have in this process of negotiation? I think that's a very open question. We haven't been training physicians for long, protracted, consensual negotiating types of decision making and we are in for a hard time as a result.

Response

C. ROLLINS HANLON, M.D.

I think what we're talking about here is the psychological aspect of relationships between an organization such as a hospital and a group of people within it. The house officers in Dr. Thompson's paper in St. Thomas' were paid a salary for partial work; the house officers in my time were paid nothing for total work. I come at this question from that kind of perspective. I come at it also with a simplified notion of hospital administration. The hospital was a much simpler thing in the thirties and forties.

I have some disagreement with Dr. Thompson, particularly where he said, "The *Darling* decision clearly closed the era of nonconcern of the board for quality of care." I think that hospital boards of trustees clearly had a concern, both for litigation and for the quality of care. It seems to me it was always concerned about people who were under the thumb of the hospital doing right. What *Darling* did, as I understand it, was to make the trustees concerned about their legal and other responsibilities for non-employees. If that person was assigned to duty in the emergency room, was he an employee or was it a *respondeat superior* situation for him as a free, independent agent?

Most of us have tended to think, if we think in adversarial terms, of hospital management staff as somewhat adversarial, and we think of the board of trustees as a referee, although, when the chips are down, the board clearly has to side with management.

Discussion

MR. JACK SHELTON: When we look back on how we got here, we shouldn't forget the role that management and labor have played. The benefits that came out of the negotiation process and the tax structure that sheltered them helped to create the structure we see today. If that structure is to change, management and labor will have to play important roles in the reshaping.

DR. JOHN A. D. COOPER: I think both Dr. Thompson and the subsequent speakers left us about ten years ago. They keep talking about a medical-social institution, but the focus now is on entrepreneurship and on business enterprise. We have a system in which physicians and hospitals are losing their unique relationships with society. Instead, they are becoming parts of a large business enterprise. I think that this change is going to have an even greater effect on what is happening than the things that the previous speakers have outlined.

I agree with Dr. Stevens that we are going to witness a shifting partnership and a shifting alliance because the whole setting in which physicians and hospitals operate is being radically changed.

DR. RICHARD S. WILBUR: I'd like to expand on a thought that Dr. Stevens expressed: the existence of a third factor besides the board of trustees and physicians. There are a great many other factors that led us to where we are. (I am assuming that where we are is in a situation in which hospitals are really too expensive for us to maintain under the current system.) These other factors are all of the other people who work in the hospitals who did not work in them under the simpler systems that evolved from Lister on: the nonphysicians and the nonmanagement. Many of them are technicians who generate enormous costs; others are those who help: the nurses, janitors, and others. As we try to put the genie back in the bottle, one of the many problems we will face is that we're not the only players in the game. There are doctors, management, boards of trustees, and an enormous supporting cast that has come to depend upon the hospital system for its economic justification.

DR. ELI GINZBERG: Since we're figuring out how we got here, I would like to make a point that hasn't been accentuated yet. This country is unique in how much it will pay in order to avoid government action, and we have been very opposed to a national health system. We didn't move to get the government into this affair until we actually had to, with Medicare, and at that point the president of the United States made a deal that is now getting unraveled; that is, he tried to make peace with the AMA by saying, "We'll put the government money in, but we won't change anything else." Well, that's what is getting unraveled now.

You can't get over 90 percent of a hospital's expenditures paid for by a third party without the third party playing a growing role in hospital affairs. I'm surprised it took nineteen years to unravel. I would have expected that to happen within five or six years, but it didn't because we were in a big expansion. I think we must go back to the very fundamental and simple matter that by the time you start to spend $150 billion a year on your hospitals, you cannot be quite using, in Dr. Cooper's terms, the old system. It's just impossible. You cannot change the whole financing area on the left and leave everything on the right untouched.

MR. PAUL ROGERS: The whole public conception has changed since the time when doctors did charity work. Since we put in Medicare and Medicaid, so that everyone expects doctors to be paid for everything, we don't expect the charity approach. The whole concept of the nonprofit nature of hospitals has also changed, and we now have for-profit hospitals. The hospital is being seen more as a business now, and we don't expect charity work or the nonprofit approach. Instead, the public is starting now to put the pressure on, to say, "You're for-profit, you're a business, let's see some results!"

PROFESSOR ALAIN ENTHOVEN: As I read Dr. Thompson's paper I was very struck when he talked about the medical staff being concerned with quality but not supposed to know anything about costs while the boards are supposed to know everything about costs but not anything about quality. There is a very strong similarity to the Defense Department which I joined in 1961 in which the military was supposed to have complete province over military requirements, strategy, forces, practices, and so forth and be absolutely unconcerned about costs. On the other hand, civilians were supposed to know all about the budget and have absolutely no involvement in strategies, forces, or practices. In fact, the Armed Services Committee wanted to pass an amendment to the law to make sure that the financial people didn't dabble in any military aspects of defense. It sort of argues with the case that each group knew the information in its power and wanted to preserve the purity of its own expertise beyond the reach of other professional groups.

I think in both cases the results were unbalanced programs with large gaps in effectiveness combined with budget overruns and waste. What we felt was needed then, which is a precursor of what's going to be coming in health care now, was a reform of financial management systems so that we could link forces to expenditures, rather like the DRG system. This approach would allow us to get ourselves in a position where we could look at cost effectiveness and at alternatives and evaluate them.

Eventually what happened is that the military had either to become cost-conscious or else to abdicate control of the military programs to civilians.

As in the defense arena twenty or twenty-five years ago, in health care now we are going to need a new class of experts: people who understand the linkage between financial and medical data. They must be able to evaluate the costs and effectiveness of alternatives, and to do policy analysis and cost-effectiveness studies.

PROFESSOR JOSEPH LIPSCOMB: I agree that there has been tension between the physicians and the hospitals over the years, but I think the case can be made that we are at a new crossroads. I think it will show itself in the kinds of tensions that will emerge as physicians and hospitals try to negotiate their own relationships. Tension seems to be a fundamental economic result from the cost control side and demand side and also from the supply and increase side, and those two types of fundamental forces ought to change the physician-hospital relationship.

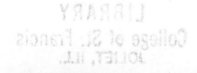

PROFESSOR THOMPSON: In the last part of my paper I hinted that these two groups, the board of trustees and the medical staff, lack a common language and consequently they were, as Dr. Enthoven said, hiding their own knowledge and their own data from each other.

The main breakthrough in diagnosis-related groups (DRGs), if indeed there is one, is the combination of fiscal and medical information in one record. That's what a DRG is.

My problem with the "new management"—and I was running a hospital when all this new management was new—is that they were managing the wrong thing! They were not helping physicians manage patient care.

My main thesis is that the old structure has to end. Both fiscal affairs and patient care are going to have to come under much closer examination by boards of trustees.

3

Physicians and Hospitals:
Tensions in the Relationship

DAVID M. KINZER

What follows is an article I wrote twenty-five years ago entitled: "The Only Team That Pilots—and Doctors—Recognize Is Their Own." The piece appeared in *The Modern Hospital*, a now-defunct hospital journal.

During World War II, I flew in the Navy off aircraft carriers. We were called the air group. It included three squadrons—fighters, dive bombers, and torpedo bombers. The squadrons broke down into wings, then divisions, and then sections. The two-plane section was the smallest unit of aerial command.

All of this was laid out neatly on the organizational chart. Within the squadron the line stairstepped up to the squadron commander, or skipper, who reported to the air group commander. The air group commander's line stretched horizontally, then vertically without break up to the executive officer and captain of the ship. In other words, the air group was on a line with all the other command departments of the ship—navigation, operations, engineering, gunnery, and air. The air department, as distinguished from the air group, was responsible for all the services and maintenance of aircraft. It should be noted that the air officer, with responsibility for the planes, and the air group commander, with responsibility for the pilots, were equals in the line of command, with neither in a position to order the other around.

Looking at the organizational chart, you would say at once that this was the orthodox line and staff organization, and that the air group was an integrated, functioning unit of the ship. There was plenty of evidence to indicate that the high Navy brass of those days thought so too.

But this was another organizational chart that concealed much more than it revealed. The group most responsible for divorcing it from reality was the pilots.

This chart was one of the things, among many others, the pilots of those days labeled as "strictly oatmeal."

We knew, you see, that this was *our* ship. It had been created for us. Obviously, therefore, the officers and crew of the ship were in our service. If they weren't they belonged on shore. In our minds, these points were beyond argument, as changeless as revealed truth. We weren't helping the ship carry out its mission; the ship helped us carry out ours. After all, what good was an aircraft carrier without pilots?

Does this sound like anything you've heard before?

We weren't at all impressed by the ship's organization, probably because we rarely thought of it as such. To us it was a place to land, a kind of floating service center where all the details incidental to our missions were accomplished. The ship therefore had to gear itself to us. The ones that accommodated themselves to us most swiftly and efficiently were the best ships.

The fact that they all made a try at doing this only served to confirm our point that the chart was just another piece of Navy paper. With the pilots' interests in mind, the Navy had applied an overlay of special privilege that almost concealed the ship's formal organization. For instance, our ready rooms were the only spaces aboard with air conditioning, except for the captain's quarters. A meal was always available to us, but not to other officers, on the off hours. We were the only ones who could get legal "drinking whiskey." A pony bottle of brandy, a good jolt, was served up to us after each strike.

We were the only officers who weren't obliged to stand a ship's watch. The ship's day was split into equal segments, and its officers and crew were parceled out so that the ship's operations were fully covered at all hours. But our day was not the ship's day. It was never that predictable. They couldn't occupy us with routines, because we had to be ready to scramble for our planes on very short notice. So we did a lot of waiting. Often we did our waiting in the sack in wardroom cabins. That was another privilege. If a pilot was found in the prone position during general quarters, it was because he was tired. Any other officer so occupied would have been up for court martial. The pilots, in fact, could be counted on to break even the most rational of Navy regulations with regularity. We were unquestionably the sloppiest group aboard ship. Anyone who had seen a Navy crew at sea knows this is quite a distinction. It used to amuse us when a senior career officer would suddenly be confronted with one of our unkempt and unshaven pilots. He would turn his head, pretending he hadn't seen him, and walk the other way.

We were convinced, though, that the privileges of perpetual readiness were more than offset by the responsibilities. Sometimes it meant taking off so late we had to land by night, or else taking off so early that we had no horizon as we mushed off the end of the deck. Sometimes it meant long stretches of furious, rushing activity without sleep. The hard part about these periods and what made them so exhausting was that, all the way through, we never felt we could let ourselves make a mistake.

While we were never happy about this aspect of the carrier pilot's life, we were, to the last man, proud of it. This, we were convinced, was the ultimate reason why we were set apart (and above) the ship's organization. The rest of the ship, we said, was geared to the clock; we were geared to the demands of our calling.

And doesn't this have a slightly familiar ring, too?

From our first days as cadets the unique status of pilots was drummed into us. Though the Navy had put us on a salary, we were appeased by flight pay, which gave us 50 percent more money than anyone else of equal rank or grade. Our appetites were whetted by a big publicity program. Pilots were made the personification of a mighty and air-minded Navy. When the press agents wrote about great victories, it was the pilot who sank the ship or shot down five of the enemy in one dogfight. They didn't bother too much about the guy who had loaded the guns.

The publicity also stressed that Navy cadets were the few chosen from the many. Even when selection standards had to be relaxed, they publicly held to this line. It not only had recruitment value; it was also designed to motivate the fledgling pilot himself. They had to make us feel privileged and select to make us equal to the kind of training program they had laid out.

They really put it to us. We had to learn jujitsu and trigonometry and other subjects that later seemed only remotely related to the business of carrier aviation. The discipline was sadistic. Even the enlisted men abused us. The one overriding objective seemed to be the shattering of our confidence.

In the early stages, our flight instructors usually told us frankly that we were hopeless. Each additional instructional period was granted as if it were a reprieve from ultimately certain execution. Once we got to the point where we could do a fairly decent landing or loop, then they'd start telling us that just learning how to fly didn't mean we could make the grade as a Navy pilot. Flying the airplane was only about 50 percent of it. The remainder was, as one of them put it, "dedication." We had to want to do it, because even in the fleet no one could really make us do what had to be done. As they put it, we were the ones, the only ones, who could "deliver the goods."

There was one instructor in particular, a tough old flying chief from the peacetime fleet, who terrorized everyone. He used to ask us technical questions on the engine or the guns that weren't even covered in the curriculum. When we couldn't answer them, he was off on a tirade about the new generation of pilots. The moral of his story was that you couldn't count on any mechanic or plane handler to do anything right unless you knew what "right" was and made sure they knew it. "Don't trust the ship too much, Sonny," he would say. "It isn't your damn mother." He washed out more of us than any other instructor. Flying ability seemed to have little to do with it. The cocky ones or the casual ones had the most trouble with him.

The training period was an eternity of torture. In no time, it had almost erased our lazy and carefree pasts from memory. The only direction we could see was ahead. Dangling on the horizon were a pair of Navy wings, which not only had become a symbol of nearly impossible attainment but were, like the flight pay, a perquisite in themselves. After all, who else but pilots could wear wings?

When we finally did make it, we had become so single-minded about our ultimate position and function that all our other "selves" were nearly invisible. There was not the slightest doubt in our minds about what we were. We were Navy pilots, members of a tight and united community of Navy pilots, the most select, the most promising, the most needed, the most God-gifted of all men.

And who else is so jazzed up after they get out of school?

All through flight training, the buildup was, "when you get into a squadron" and "when the squadron gets to the fleet." There was almost nothing said about the ship itself and how we fitted in. So when we got our ship and landed aboard one day, we amazed and shocked the crew with our inclusive ignorance of ship routines and organization.

The ship was enormous, a maze of technology, a honeycomb of specialization. At first we couldn't even find our way around, not to mention understanding what all the paraphernalia was, what it was for, the voluminous edicts governing its use, who uses it, the protocol involved, and so on. Actually our initial curiosity was blunted by the incredible complexity of everything.

This feeling of strangeness, which lasted for many weeks, had the effect of drawing us even more closely together. We felt like a small minority and we were. There were literally thousands of enlisted men carrying out specialized and often incomprehensible assignments—mechanics and radiomen and ordnance men, each group broken down into numerous specialties and subspecialties, the men who fixed and calibrated the radar, others who operated it, others who interpreted it. Besides the ship's radar, each plane type used a different type of radar, each with its own maintenance specialist.

There was no end to it. On the flight deck there were hook disengagers, wing folders, taxi signalers, radio checkers, instrument checkers, firemen, crashmen, corpsmen, and signalmen.

The Navy had started years before sending these people to special schools. They were coming aboard ship with a specialty as well as a rating. On their sleeves they proudly wore the emblems of their attainment. Some of them even wore their own special kind of wings. When the Navy started doing this, the pilots made outraged protests. "Sure," we'd say, "we grant you that they deserve recognition, but this is confusing to the public. They'll think these guys are flying the damn airplanes."

Meet the "parapilots."

Their specialization notwithstanding, to us this array of highly trained technicians was still an amorphous mass we called "the crew." Even after months, there were few that we even recognized, not to speak of knowing them as individuals. They lived in a different world, statuswise and timewise. We always said to ourselves that we should make an effort to know them, but there never seemed to be the time. There were pilots who went through a whole tour of duty without being able to identify some of the insignia they wore on their sleeves.

We knew the ship's officers better, since the Navy had made us equals in wardroom society. But that didn't mean we felt close to them. Partly it was because we had our own language. It was much easier just to talk to each other. Partly, but only partly, it was a matter of status, symbolized by the wings we wore on our shirts.

The latter point must be carefully qualified. The ship's captain, the exec, and the air officer had wings, too, but that didn't mean they were in the brotherhood. They disqualified themselves on two counts: one, they were not actually flying with us (few command officers ever left the deck), and, two, they were hopelessly and irrevocably organization men, at once the spokesmen and the servants of the ship. Among ourselves, we didn't consider them fliers at all.

Even squadron skippers were on trial until they established their loyalties one way or another. What we expected from them was steady and predictable leadership in the air, which implied a pretty fair competence as an aviator, and a readiness to go to bat for their pilots in any and all situations that involved a conflict with the ship.

Whether by brilliance or accident, the Navy did very well in its selection of squadron commanders. I never ran into a really bad one. They had an uncanny knack of picking men with absolutely no administrative abilities whatsoever and only the dimmest of ambitions for a postwar Navy career. This was exactly what the pilots wanted. The administrator type was, by definition, not air-minded; the ambitious would inevitably cozy up to the high rank on board and try to sell us an organization bill of goods.

In short, there was a pretty clear line that cut across the officers' wardroom. There were the guys who flew the planes and there were the "gumshoes," our word for the guys who didn't fly the planes. I can recall our making only two exceptions to this social line of distinction. One was the landing signal officer. He had to be one of us because it was a psychological necessity that we trust him completely. The other was the flight surgeon. He earned his wings when he sold the captain on giving us the brandy.

Which should establish, if we have not already done so, that pilots and doctors are very close together in their basic thinking.

One thing the pilots all learned quickly was that spectacular success and complete disaster were always uncomfortably close companions. The first could rarely be realized without the near presence of the other. In fighters it was that extra 100 or 200 yards of pressing in close on an enemy plane. In dive bombers it was maybe about 1,000 more feet of waiting to be sure before you pressed the release button. This, we assumed, was what our instructors had meant by "dedication," because this was the part that nobody could ever really make us do.

The fact that they couldn't make us do it put us under more of a strain, I think, than there might have been otherwise. Nobody was ever enthusiastic about being bracketed by a hail of small caliber fire near the ground or close to an enemy formation. Some days, though, we were less enthusiastic than others. Day by day, in other words, we fought a running battle with ourselves about just how hard a try we would give it. Aside from the willpower factor, there was a fine point of judgment. We had to know when success was impossible, when the real hard try was suicide and a waste, when it would be wiser to come back and try another day. In spite of what the publicists said, these choices were often possible. Every pilot who lived through the war made them prudently.

This probably explains why the pilots, of all the groups on ship, were the least inclined toward open criticism of their fellows. The word of someone's conspicuous aerial failure stayed within the group. Usually we tried to make it easier for the man involved. All of us had failed on occasions, too.

If we ever heard another pilot's performance being criticized by a ship's officer or crew member, we rammed the words right back down their throats. It was very important to us that this kind of thing not be accepted, or even acknowledged.

At the heart of this ethic was a deep sense that no outsider could possibly appreciate what we were going through. Given this, we didn't grant any right of criticism.

So, mixed in with our pride was a chronic inner discomfort. We had a responsibility. There was no limit to it. So we had to do the limiting ourselves. What we did in the air war and the inner war that went with it completely wrapped us up. This was our nagging preoccupation, even when we weren't flying. This was what was important.

I try to explain this feeling because it in turn explains why the pilots drew such a clear line between themselves and the ship and why we were so suspicious of anyone whose primary interests lay with the ship's organization. They did not and they could not understand that our problems were always more important to us than any the ship could give us.

We wanted the ship to leave us alone with our problems. In return we were glad to let the captain and all his crew have theirs.

But it didn't work out that way. The ship had to involve itself in our problems because, as they put it, we were a part of the ship. For identical reasons, they argued that we should help the ship solve its problems, too.

As you can see, "togetherness" was a common theme in those days, too.

There was an unremitting, obsessive, and ceaselessly inventive effort to get the pilots "on the team." It came at us like a crossfire from many levels of the Navy hierarchy, from the task force right up to Washington. On the ship there was always someone from air plot, the flight deck, maintenance, or air intelligence who sought and obtained an audience with the pilots to get their "cooperation and understanding" in the solution of some "mutual problem." We were beset by an endless stream of directives, reports, instructions, and other paper from Washington. Nearly every month the high brass changed its mind on how we should fly the airplane.

Not content with just educating us, the Navy had to study, test, and evaluate us, too. In the later stages of the war, sociologists, psychologists, and an assortment of other obscure functionaries in the human relations field began to close in on us. The word had gotten out and up, you see, that the pilots were "a problem" all through the fleet. One central thesis had apparently won full acceptance—that if someone could just figure out a way to build an identity of interest between pilot and ship the war would quickly be won.

Our response to all of this wasn't exactly gratifying to the Navy. The pressure seemed to create its own resistance. Being preoccupied, we were easily bored with this kind of attention. Besides we quickly found that about half the ideas they had for us didn't work. You don't teach anybody to dogfight an F6F at 30,000 feet by writing a memo and holding a meeting, but these things were tried. We went to the meetings sure that none of the ideas was any good.

Sometimes it got so heavy that whole squadrons would work themselves into a kind of frenzy. "Why don't they leave us alone," we would ask each other, "and spend their time learning how to keep the damn canopies clean."

The canopies were a chronic and apparently insoluble problem. I once had four planes at a stretch that had an oil glaze on the windbreak front of the canopies. Obviously we couldn't sight very well on a target with oil distorting the image.

Getting the windshields cleaned properly was a problem. We'd ask the plane captain why he hadn't cleaned it, and he'd say he had. And we'd say that it wasn't clean, and he'd admit it wasn't.

And then we'd tell him that the way to get oil off glass was to use a gasoline-soaked rag, and he knew that, too. And then he'd tell us his problem. There was an order against using gasoline-soaked rags on the flight decks with engines turning up. Then we'd ask why they hadn't cleaned it down in the hangar deck, and he didn't know. Besides it wasn't his responsibility. He was a plane captain, not a mechanic.

This upset me so much that I actually tried to find the man responsible for keeping that canopy clean. There wasn't a sailor on that ship, though, who would admit a responsibility for any-thing except in the physical presence of his chief petty officer. The chiefs, of course, were the unrivaled masters of self-absolution. Nothing was ever their fault. So you and your problem would land with some ship's officer, who didn't know the culprit either. It annoyed him to be asked because, as he put it, the chief handled all such details.

Besides those of us who were sore about dirty canopies, there were other pilots ranging furiously up and down the ship trying to find who had fouled up their guns or had forgotten to bolt down their engine housing or had reversed the wires on their ele-vator trim. If all of this accomplished nothing else, we did shake the chain of command from the bottom up and antagonized many an innocent member of the crew.

This got to such a point on one ship that the air officer called us together and told us in no uncertain terms to lay off his en-listed men. Then he announced with evident pride that he had a solution to the problem. From that time on, we were to channel our complaints through junior officers who had been assigned to each squadron just for that purpose.

Looking back over the years, the plight of these commissioned "troubleshooters" inspires pity; at the time, though, we felt no charity and gave no mercy. From the very start, their jobs were a nightmare. They took the full brunt of every complaint that we had and some that we imagined. Often they didn't swing enough weight with the chiefs and the maintenance crews to get action. Often part of the message was lost in transmittal. Often it wasn't understood in the first place. Of course, they always got it worse from us the second time around when we discovered the thing never was fixed.

The failures of these three helpless ensigns confirmed the very darkest misgivings we had about administrative officers. They seemed to know everything but how to give us fast and dependable service. In the privacy of our ready rooms we delivered this unanimous verdict: They were "meddlers, bunglers, fools."

In how many doctors' lounges have these kind of cries resounded?

We soon had the feeling that nobody on the ship liked us. Walking along the catwalks on our way to the plane, we'd often hear profane mutterings from members of the crew—loud enough to get the sense of but never clear enough for positive identification. In their own ways the ship's officers made their feelings clear, too.

But though it was true that the ship wasn't very happy about us, it wasn't very happy about anything else, either. I was on four carriers during the war—one ship that was very good, two ships that were average, and one ship that was terrible. All of the ships were unhappy.

The reasons this was so are complex but familiar. Bigness had blighted the personal touch and thereby made communication difficult. People didn't feel like "shipmates" when they didn't see one another from one month to the next. There was some departmental esprit, but it often had its outlet in vindictiveness against the men in other departments. So there were eternal little wars being fought within the big war.

The Navy had passed out so many ranks and grades in so many specialties that there was a terrible status problem. They had a hard enough time even finding a place to put some of these people in the organizational structure. Making them feel that they fitted was a problem that few had time to tackle. The pilots weren't the only ones who had gotten specialized training and a buildup that made them feel the ship couldn't exist without them. It seemed like half the people aboard had had more or less the same experience. Everybody had his letdown, too.

So the pilots were not the only ones aboard that ship who were resented. In fact, we probably ranked a poor third behind the captain and the cooks. Resentments flowed up and down and across every line of the ship's organization, but they did tend to concentrate more on symbols than on personalities. The captain symbolized authority, the pilots symbolized special privilege, and the cooks symbolized food. On Navy ships, nobody ever liked any of these things.

In other words, the crew had to complain. It was a universal compulsion. In this respect the pilots were very much a part of the ship's organization, never lacking contribution to the general chorus. For one thing, we were mad about the rule that permitted brandy only if we had been in actual combat with the enemy; our contention was that you needed it just as much after searches or combat air patrols when you could have been shot at and were fully expecting to be shot at almost any time.

Maybe 70 percent of all the resentments and complaints were pointed in the general direction of the ship's captain. The foregoing complaint is a good example. Since we couldn't blame an unenlightened brandy policy on anyone else (the flight surgeon had tried hard), we had to blame it on the captain. Take all the specialized groups on that ship, multiply that by all the specialized interests they were trying to promote, and consider that most of these issues either would not or could not be resolved and would therefore be raised at least once a day every day at sea, and then you can understand why the captain spent so much time alone in his cabin.

There is much more that I could say about the aircraft carrier and its pilots. This should be enough, though, to cast serious doubts on the common assumption that the stresses and strains in the relationship of medical staff to the hospital organization, and vice versa, are absolutely unique, and that we can therefore get little help or solace from looking at the experience in other fields.

Having had a few years to mull all of this over, I can state with some assurance the following conclusions—about pilots and aircraft carriers, of course—but hoping, in the process, to stir up some good arguments about their application to hospitals and doctors.

1. The conflict between pilot and carrier would have persisted in any kind of organizational structure. Note that the Navy had denied the pilots any semblance of the functional authority that the physician has when he directs patient care activities within the hospital. There were no dotted lines for us. We had our place in the line of command, just like the others. But the Navy did not, by virtue of this decision, make us organization-minded or even eliminate the ambivalence and confusion that is so often noted in the hydra-headed hospital organization. Fifteen years away from my experience, I feel sure (without checking myself) that the Navy still hasn't solved this "problem."

2. Strains in the pilot-carrier relationship stemmed from a functional conflict, and not a conflict that derived from weakness in the ship's organization. The pilots were, and had to be, individ-

ualized and independent in their approach to their responsibilities; the carrier, by equivalent necessity, had to press constantly for conformity. A kind of uneasy equilibrium of these opposing forces had to be maintained. The process of maintaining this equilibrium went on outside the framework of shipboard authority and organization.

3. The pilots had to be aggressive, had to act like they had authority over the organization, in order to keep this balance. It comes back to the basic question of who else the ship was serving but us. We had to keep reminding them that it was us. Otherwise the organization would have swamped us. One day we lost a pilot off the catapult. He just dribbled off and under the bow of our ship going thirty knots full tilt into the wind. Someone at some time who had had something to do with that catapult had fouled up. Our squadron skipper was unforgettable that day. First he told off the ship's captain and then went straight down the line with everybody who had even a remote connection with that catapult. He never did find out who was responsible, but we didn't have any more catapult failures on that cruise, either. In bullying and antagonizing the ship's officers and crew, we were really protecting ourselves. We were acutely conscious of the fact that the ship, just like the pilot, was capable of disastrous error. Usually these errors hurt us.

4. In spite of the pilots' sensitivity about ship domination and direction, the last thing we really wanted was authority over the ship and the responsibilities attached thereto. Long before, the Navy had decided that this wouldn't work. Their reasons: (a) it took too long to train good pilots who were also skilled and knowledgeable about engines and electronics and the supervision and organization of human activity. So they chose to concentrate on training good pilots; (b) the mission to be accomplished was so important that it was absolutely imperative that we be made a part of a much larger organization that keyed into large strategies and objectives; and (c) they had to free us of any distraction that might interfere with the execution of our primary function. The pilots didn't argue with this. We felt we already had enough responsibilities. As stated, what we really wanted was good service.

Granting the organization its power and influence, then we had a right to expect decisiveness from the captains and admirals who held this power in custody. In other words, the last thing we really wanted was weakness and permissiveness from the men in top command. Since no decision of any importance was easy, these men had to have courage. To make up for some of my slanderous remarks, I would like to say that the Navy had a good quota of command officers equal to these decisions. If I had the time I could tell some good stories about them. Suffice it to say that long after most of the pilots' exploits have lost shape and significance, certain command decisions still live in my book as the most heroic acts of the whole war.

The pilots would never be, and could never be, members of a Navy shipboard "team" in any literal sense. This does not imply that cooperation with the ship was not important or necessary. It means only that the effort to get us to accept a shoulder-to-shoulder relationship with the ship was representative of a kind of loose thinking in administrative circles that is so often self-defeating.

The point is this: The only real "team" relationship the pilots had was with the other pilots. This had meaning. When the fighters, dive bombers, and torpedo planes made what we called a co-ordinated attack on an enemy ship, and actually coordinated it, that was teamwork. This was something quite different from our relationship with taxi-men, wing folders, or mechanics. They had to accommodate themselves to us, like the trainer on a football team. Certainly it was important to work smoothly with them, but when they asked us to understand their problems and make their jobs easier—in the analogy, run interference for them—they were asking too much.

We were rightly suspicious of this kind of "team" talk. It is significant that it was most prevalent on the worst ships. What the men in command really were asking was for help in solving *their* problem. They had to make a complex and sometimes unwieldy organization work; it was all too easy to blame its failures on the group upon which all activities focused.

Those who spent more time coordinating and perfecting these supportive activities had far fewer problems with the pilots. This is where administrative genius could have been used to good effect but usually wasn't.

It was a good thing the admirals and the captains never occupied themselves very seriously with the problems of human relations, of making their subordinates happy with their jobs and happy with each other. If they had gotten into this problem, we'd still be trying to win the war.

To paraphrase my main point in this article I published twenty-five years ago, these tensions are built into the relationship and will not and cannot be eliminated as a cause of conflict, regardless of the efforts of the carrier—or the hospital. To quote from the article: "The pilots were, and had to be, individualized and independent in their approach to their responsibilities; the carrier, by equivalent necessity, had to press constantly for conformity. A kind of uneasy equilibrium of these opposing forces had to be maintained."

In a time when hospital-doctor relationships are a central point of concern and when the tensions relating thereto seem to be on the increase, this main point deserves elaboration.

To start with, I suggest that it is not in the interests of the hospital (or the general public) that we make members of medical staffs into "organization men," even if it were possible to do so. Just like the wartime pilots, physicians weren't trained to be "organization men." The main thrust of our pilots' training was to identify and build upon the qualities of initiative, creativity, sound judgment, and courage. Manual dexterity and coordination were important, too, but were useless attributes unless we had the others. Though the Navy imposed tight organization and discipline on its carrier air groups, we were not in any real sense "standardized."

The success or failure of our performance as pilots was measured in "one-on-one" situations. No dive bombing run on an enemy ship or dogfight with an enemy plane was like any other. It was always a very lonely experience. The carrier we took off from and, we hoped, would land back upon was always, during these moments, a remote and almost irrelevant entity. Our full attention was captured by the challenging business at hand. It was a very personal thing, which the ship had no part of. If we thought about the ship at all, it was with a nearly subconscious expectation that the ship would be where it was supposed to be (it wasn't always) when our mission was completed and we headed home.

An explicit reality here is that the mission of the pilot and the carrier were *not* the same. Nor is the mission of the hospital and the clinicians on its medical staff. This distinction is important. The carrier (or the hospital) is an organization whose only reason for being is to provide a support system for the mission of its pilots (or physicians). Whether the "mission" is a dogfight or a critical trauma case, it is still the prime responsibility of the pilot or the attending physician. The organization, with its technical hardware, supply system, and support personnel, has only a backup role.

This may seem like an extremely elementary and obvious point, except that what I am seeing and hearing a lot of nowadays stands as an impressive body of evidence that a high proportion of the professionals in our business do not understand it or accept it.

It is clear that this point is not accepted by the still proliferating number of nonmedical professionals in our hospitals. I speak here of nurses, physical therapists, psychiatric counselors, and others who continue to press for "independent functions" in direct patient care. Hospital management is exhibiting in its recent behavior some reluctance as well. Some Young Turks in hospital management seem to perceive their role to be one of "managing" medical services. This tendency is clearly being fueled by the new climate created by the DRG payment system for Medicare.

Under this new economic pressure, there is a push within hospital management to contain the initiatives of individual medical staff members within the parameters of a preset price for a diagnosis. The impulse here, and the subject of much discussion in administrative circles, is how and in what way to "discipline the outliers." In my frequent conversations with government health bureaucrats, it is apparent that many of them are rooting for this kind of administrative behavior. They don't yet know how to enforce this kind of discipline directly on the practicing physician, nor do many of them seem to want to try.

Of all the articles I have written, my "Pilots" piece has attracted the most attention. I still get requests for reprints. It seems to be most appreciated by practicing physicians, possibly because it tends to glamorize and glorify a calling that has many humdrum moments and obligations. Many of the patient problems physicians are expected to treat are about as boring and as lacking in any constructive result as some of the search missions or combat air patrols we used to have to fly when everyone was pretty sure any possible enemy was thousands of miles away.

Has time reduced the validity of my analogy, given the fact that the intervening years have brought major change to both carrier aviation and the delivery of medical services in our country? I think not. As a loyal alumnus of the Navy Air Corps, I've done my best to keep track of changes there. Going back to the post-Korean War era, I recall spending an evening with a fighter squadron commander who, after a few drinks, complained bitterly about a cost-cutting initiative of that time. Each squadron was given a monthly ration of gasoline which, if consumed too soon, meant that the squadron had to quit flying for the balance of the month. "How do they expect me to maintain a situation of readiness," he grumbled, "when my pilots can't even fly?"

And there is the story told me by one of my vice-presidents, who was a carrier-based attack plane pilot during the Vietnam War. There was a policy at that time of not allowing any of the pilots to fly below five thousand feet over enemy territory because any shrapnel that might pierce the skins of planes could cause irreparable damage to computer-packed aircraft that had already become superexpensive. "The problem was," he told me, "that we couldn't hit anything from 5,000 feet. Mostly we couldn't even see a target."

Then, just a couple of years ago, I spent some time talking things over with members of a carrier fighter group based on the USS John F. Kennedy, temporarily docked in Boston. The main lament of this group was about computers. The whole carrier, along with its planes, was computerized. In the pilots' ready room was a screen which, through computers, was supposed to convey the exact position of every airborne plane in the squadron. Except that it didn't work. There were a lot of other computers on that ship that didn't work, either. At any given time, they told me, at least half the planes in their squadron were nonoperational because of computer problems. In fact, as I was told, the planes they had could be landed aboard ship at night by computer without the pilot even needing to touch the stick. I asked the pilots whether they felt comfortable with this innovation. They all said no. I asked them if they ever used it. They all said no.

As they explained it, the problem with the computers was a problem with computer technicians. After the Navy had spent the money to train these exotic specialists and assigned them aboard ship, they were soon lured away by much higher pay in the burgeoning stateside private computer industry.

You can pick and choose from any of the above for comparisons with some of the problems confronted recently in our hospital medical practice world.

On the cost issue, there is also telling experience. The plane I flew near the war's end, the F4U4 Corsair, had a "final unit flyaway cost" of $230,000. The Navy tells me that the "flyaway cost" of its most sophisticated new aircraft, the F/A-18, is $22,858,000, or 100 times as much. In communicating this to me, the Naval public information officer felt impelled to justify the difference. "The F4U4," he said, "was a very basic fighter aircraft. The most advanced instruments in its cockpit were a radio and a primitive search finder. The F/A-18 has eleven onboard computers and two high-performance F404 engines. The F/A-18 is capable of launching nine long-range Phoenix missiles and tracking twenty-seven different targets simultaneously."

I was also told that the Essex-class carrier that I flew from in 1943 cost $55,227,944. The latest bid they have received for the next nuclear-powered CVN is $1.6 billion, almost thirty times as much. In shipbuilding, the PR specialist told me, the labor cost for one week is twenty-one times as much as in 1937.

None of this seems very different from what has happened to the cost of the support system for modern medical practice since the end of World War II.

The point in my "Pilots" piece that seems most deserving of emphasis is the need for top-level management (the ship's captain) to accept physician behavior (or pilot behavior) as one of the givens in his management equation. It is a waste of time to try to change characteristics that have been built upon all the way back to the selection and training process. The wise and effective manager is one who understands this point. "It was all too easy to blame its (i.e., the ship's) failures on the group upon which all activities focused. . . . Those who spent more time coordinating and perfecting these supportive activities had many less problems with the pilots." Also relating to present reality on our medical care scene, the good hospital CEO, like the good carrier skipper, must recognize that most of his staff physicians (or pilots) don't want to be bothered with management responsibilities, but they do expect to function in an environment that is well managed. We are hearing a lot these days about the need to bring more physicians onto the "management team." I suggest that, given the nature of the medical beast, this has only limited potential. I am not saying that all physi ians are, by definition, poor managers or that there are not some very good managers who happen to be physicians who perform well in top health care management jobs—only that getting more physicians into management has only limited potential for easing our problem of mounting tensions between hospitals and medical staffs. The real key to this is better understanding of each other's problems and diverse missions. This can only happen where there is more frequent and open dialogue between the two parties. This currently does not happen in many of our hospitals.

The boards of hospitals have a crucial role here. They, above all other involved parties, must understand the balance that needs to be maintained. On the management side, they must begin to insist on "strong" management and give more protection to its strength. This implies more delegation than we see in many hospitals, but also more definition of the parameters of administrative authority. On issues relating to medical staff, the boards can't stay out of it. They can't fairly expect their CEO to be the "hatchet man" of so-called aberrant medical staff performers. The boards have to set the standards for overall medical staff performance, and require the medical staff as a collective entity to meet these standards. This is not so much an administrative responsibility for the medical staff as it is one of collective discipline, which is what the Navy demanded of all of its carrier air groups.

I define "strong" management to mean someone who makes decisions on how the hospital must stay within forever-after-limited budget targets. This person must clearly have the capacity, with board support, to enforce these limits. But the caveat here is that he cannot be the "enforcer" on individual medical staff member performance.

On the medical staff side, there's a quid pro quo. It is one of delivering on its "accountability," once it is defined. Medical staff organizations, to quote numerous pundits, have been "useless" as an instrument for controlling expenditures and too often, of course, as an instrument for controlling quality of performance as well. On the financial side, they must be persuaded that they will be functioning within overall limits not dissimilar from those imposed upon my post-Korean War fighter squadron commander coping with gasoline rationing. They must also be persuaded that they are the main source of pressure, and constraint, on the super-expensive technological commitment of the hospital. As on my aircraft carrier, technological improvements, regardless of their costs, can no longer be acceptable as an end in themselves. The doctors have to make some important collective decisions here on what is most relevant to the improvement of services to their patients in their hospital.

In conclusion, let me offer some observations on recent changes affecting the practice of medicine in our country and on how they seem to relate to the problem of growing tensions between the physicians and their hospital (or other organized patient-care setting).

1. *Changes in mode of practice.* The solo fee-for-service office practice, an idealized model for many years, is now viewed as an anachronism by most new graduates entering practice. Mostly, they are going to work for something or somebody—a partnership, a medical group, an HMO, a hospital, or a private for-profit corporation—and often on a salaried basis. Does this change the character of the tensions I have tried to describe? Maybe a little bit, but I hope not very much. Regardless of who the doctor works for, he carries with him a primary commitment to his patients, which includes protecting those patients' welfare against any and all organizational intrusions.

2. *Ethical considerations.* The ethics of the medical profession have far more meaning and deeper historical roots than any that might be said to apply to a community hospital or its administrator or to the business ethics of a proprietary hospital corporation, an IPA, or an HMO. We are well into an era where ethics (the right to die, the defensibility of "heroic" medical interventions, "defensive medicine," etc.) has become a focus of concern for the media, the courts, the clergy, politicians, and a very involved public. But who is in the best position to decide what is "right" for the patient and his concerned family? A difficult question nowadays, but I suggest that, if the physician backs away from his central position in this decision-making process, he abrogates one of his most important responsibilities. More than ever before, the hospital as an entity is implicated in this process. In the interest of maintaining organizational-medical balance inside the hospital, it is in everyone's interest that the hospital sustain the physician's central role in this decision-making process.

3. *The oversupply of physicians.* In many areas of the country the growing abundance of licensed practitioners is tipping the balance of power to the organizations that increasingly "deliver" the bulk of medical services in our country. These organizations, importantly including hospitals, are moving into a "buyer's market" in their contracting or other arrangements for medical services. "Closed staff" has become a subject at the hospital board level. So has setting "conditions" for renewing staff appointments, such as requiring that appointees admit patients exclusively to that hospital and not become involved in competing "freestanding" laboratories or surgicenters or ambulatory care outreach centers on the side. This is an area where increasing

tension seems guaranteed, and where the maximum of understanding and free give-and-take dialogue is needed.

4. *The "freestanding" issue.* The proliferating number of "surgicenters," "urgicenters," "emergicenters," and other "doc-in-a-box" operations is of course a spillout result of the growing abundance of physicians referred to above. This competitive initiative seems unstoppable, especially when the only control on it is medical licensure. It only becomes a source of tension when the medical entrepreneurs behind these enterprises are competing with the hospitals where they hold admitting privileges. There is a simple answer to this one—it is a free country and medicine is still a free profession but, soon enough, the doctors involved should be required to make a choice, one or the other. The oversupply situation is moving us inexorably toward two kinds of medical practice, hospital-based and "other." More hospital selectivity seems indicated in any case, given the ridiculously bloated size of many of the medical staffs of our community hospitals, dimensions that make it nearly impossible to establish staff accountability to the hospital. It would be like letting any pilot who had a license and an interest join our carrier air group. What I am trying to suggest is that limiting the size of a staff and clearly defining hospital expectations of that staff will achieve more over time in relieving tensions than will increasing staff size. When the distinctions between hospital and nonhospital medical practice are more clearly defined, I don't have any worries about which will win the competition for talent. In my analogy, the "freestandings" look like a bunch of privateers trying to get in on a war the carriers and battleships are already positioned to fight.

5. *The cost issue.* To date the mandate for controlling costs and the risks for failing to control them mostly has been laid upon our hospitals. To an amazing degree, physicians have not viewed hospital costs as *their* problem. But, as more and more states install global limits on hospital revenues, this lack of concern or commitment can't be allowed to go on much longer. In Massachusetts, where global limits on hospital revenues are a new and uncomfortable reality, we are now in the awkward position of having economic incentives in hospital payment that openly conflict with the economic incentives of fee-for-service medical practice. Here is another source of building tension. In my Naval air analogy, it would be like the pilots not caring in wartime whether the government was appropriating enough money to buy airplanes and aircraft carriers.

6. *The "charity-care" issue.* The "unsponsored" caseload seeking care in our hospitals continues to mount in many areas of our country. As governments, federal and state, cut back on their payment and coverage commitments, the affected public still expects to receive essential medical services from community hospitals and their medical staffs. Here is another area of mounting tension between hospitals and their staffs. How can a hospital maintain its "charitable" standing, in legal terms and in terms of sustaining its local public service image, when its own staff physicians refuse to take care of poor people and sometimes even patients who are on Medicaid? On this issue, it has become impossible to separate the interests of the hospital and its medical staff. It would be like a carrier sortie to intercept an enemy task force when the air group refuses to take off from the ship.

7. *The push for more cost control.* Finally, the main point of emphasis. The most powerful force that is building hospital-medical staff tensions is the push for more cost control. It is coming at us from all directions. It is the most difficult one of all to deal with, given what I have described as the temptations it puts on health care managers to apply normative pressures on the practice of medicine. I believe that one of the solemn obligations of hospitals and similar institutions in these times is to preserve and protect the discretion of their physicians to do their utmost for each of their patients, regardless of the ultimate cost. We should never forget that some of our very best physicians are "aberrant performers." Our whole system builds from the one-on-one doctor-patient covenant. If this is much abridged or diminished, we lose a lot. I worry especially about what the new normative pressures might do to medical practice inside our great medical centers, where creative innovation is a priceless ingredient.

All of the above notwithstanding, the obligation to protect the professional prerogatives of individual physicians must be related to the reality that, soon enough, all of our hospitals will be forced to live with preset limitations on their revenue or expense. Soon enough there will certainly be new constraints on how much physicians can charge, at least for government-sponsored patients. There is even consideration of imposing aggregate limitations on billings from both hospitals and their medical staffs. In this environment, the options will be closer cooperation or warfare. It is hard to see how this can come out anywhere in between.

The question is not whether costs will be controlled, but how.

The physicians must be involved in this decision-making process. At the hospital level, I think it will be the wisest course to make these decisions around what services should or should not be provided, or around the volume limits of a given service that will be delivered, rather than setting any limit on how much service an individual physician can deliver to his patient. This would be like trying to tell one of our ace Navy fighter pilots how many times he's allowed to fire at the enemy.

Response

J. ALEXANDER MCMAHON

I think it is high time that we reanalyze the relationships between the various players in the hospital, a subject that the officers of the American Hospital Association and the American Medical Association devoted a great deal of time to in their last meeting.

We have a new day: a new day of cost constraints; a new day of number of physicians; to some extent a new day in the growth of technology; certainly a new day with respect to equity in ethical issues that are coming down the track.

I think we owe Mr. Kinzer a great debt for the wartime carrier analogy that he used. Certainly, it is better than the three-legged stool; certainly, it adds a greater dimension than the doctor's workshop; and it may even be better than my own analogy. I spoke to the management group at Duke University some years ago and drew an analogy between the hospital and the university. Both have boards. Both have administrations. One has a faculty and one has a medical staff. One has students, the other has patients. One has alumni and the other has a community to serve. The analogy, as I have pondered it over the years, does not give a great deal of hope to hospitals, but it may give us all the comfort of not being alone.

One place I had a little difficulty with Mr. Kinzer's analogy is that the carrier and the naval air group had a mission given to them: to search out a Japanese carrier group and destroy it. This is a simplification, of course, of what was going on in the ship, but the strategy was given as were the tactical concerns. They didn't need a board because the mission was known.

On the other hand, a hospital, including its medical staff, has to define its own mission. Sometimes there are some givens, such as a role to play in medical education. There wouldn't be a need for a hospital if it weren't part of the educational mission of the university. So, the key role of the institution, including the medical staff, is to come to its own definition of mission because it is not going to be given any strategic missions from the outside.

It seems to me clearly that the survival of hospitals and the physicians who are intensely dependent on it lies in rethinking the relationship between those two factors, not in reducing the tension. An institution without any constructive tension probably isn't going anyplace. It is only when there is movement that tension develops and that's the reason it is time for us to be rethinking intrahospital relationships.

I close with the good news and the bad news. The good news is that something is happening. There has been a remarkable reduction in the rate of increase in hospital costs however you look at it: total cost, cost per case, cost per day; and the trend line continues to point downward. I'm not sure why that is so but if you look at the three-month period ending in November 1983—before DRGS got in place—the Fiscal Responsibility Act enacted in August of 1982 had already begun to affect relationships. So, the good news is that things are coming down, and coming down rapidly enough so that we no longer have to think of draconian measures of reducing hospital costs. What we now have to do is to improve the system already headed in the right direction in order to avoid dramatic or traumatic changes.

Now, the bad news is that the improvement in costs cannot be clearly ascribed to better relationships across the board.

H. L. Mencken once said, "To every complex issue, there is a solution that's direct, simple, and wrong." As we grope toward a better understanding of hospital relationships, let us not take simplistic solutions.

Response

JAMES H. SAMMONS, M.D.

I think Mr. Kinzer's analogy is absolutely superb. I have known very few pilots and absolutely no doctors who were not totally individualistic.

One of the disturbing things that Mr. Kinzer addressed in his paper is that we are in danger of forgetting the ethical implications of all the things that are happening. As I travel around the country today, for the first time ever I see a level of physician anxiety that I have never seen before. It borders on an even worse paranoia than there was in the early sixties when the debate was raging on Medicare and Medicaid. It is a much greater fear of what is presumed to be unknown, and that unknown is the relationship that doctors will have with the institutions in which they work and the people with whom they work, and the patients on whom they work.

The federal government is responsible in great part for having produced it. The DRG concept has brought with it a great anxiety about the ability of the individual physician to practice and to treat patients as they need to be and should be treated. I think Mr. Kinzer recognizes that. He says that the prime obligation of the hospital is to ensure freedom of the physician to continue to treat his or her patients. Whether that will work or not remains to be seen.

I read an article the other day that was written back in the early fifties in which the author was talking about physician ownership of hospitals. He made the observation at the end that in his opinion that's the way it should have been in the fifties. What happened between the fifties and the eighties is the doctors quit owning and operating hospitals. There are some doctors who are good managers, but most doctors are good doctors and not good managers. Most hospital administrators are good managers and not doctors. That thirty-odd-year transition from the marginal hospitals that were doctor-owned or doctor-monopolized to big institutions with a relatively impersonal management approach has enhanced the high levels of anxiety that we see in this country today.

I think that we really are at the crossroads. And I wonder what the future relationship of doctors and hospital administrations will be down the road. You cannot have physicians who become total managers. On the other hand, I would fight to the bloody death in the absolute belief that unless doctors become active as part of the hospital board or management in some fashion, the gulf will widen, levels of suspicion will increase, and the amount of misunderstanding will grow.

One of the things that Mr. Kinzer addresses and then leaves rather quickly is the increasing number of physicians in this country. I think more needs to be said about this than just the simple observation that the increasing number of physicians is itself creating a high level of anxiety. It represents a competitive aspect in the face of reduced expenditures and an effort to reduce them more than this profession has ever seen. This is the first time in the history of this country that anybody has ever attempted to put the brakes on what was being spent for health and medical care for Americans. We went through the steak and salad days so fast that many of us didn't believe that the steak would ever run out. It did, suddenly, and we were confronted with a whole new series of problems, not the least of which is the rate of production of physicians in this country. I am more concerned about what that means in terms of quality of medical care than I am in terms of its impact on the physician-hospital relationship. I think we all have to address both aspects, however, because there is going to be a great deal of "shopping around" by hospital administrations and it's going to be in both the proprietary and the nonproprietary sense.

I do wish we could stop talking about these two hospital systems as though they were on different planets because they're not. The same factors that drive the proprietary hospitals to make a profit drive the not-for-profits to make a profit. The sooner we all recognize that we're talking about all hospitals and not one group or the other, the sooner we can come to some kind of consensus as to how they should be handled.

We are going to see a lot of "shopping around" by hospital administrations for physicians who will fit a mold. Not every hospital administrator in the country is going to be prepared to ensure that the institution provides freedom for the physician to practice. Not every hospital administrator in the country is going to spend a lot of time worrying about what happens to the quality of care in that institution. The big worry for the administrator is a satisfactory bottom line on the profit and loss statement at the end of the year, so that he or she can go to the board of trustees and say, "Well, we don't have to have a fund drive of the magnitude we had last year!" or "I don't have to go back to First City and borrow another twenty million dollars!"

The fact that there is a very high production of physicians on an annual basis simply helps drive that machine. I'm not suggesting any kinds of arbitrary or artificial limits on the production of physicians. It is the AMA's often-stated point of view that the decision about the size of medical school classes rests precisely where it belongs: in the hands of the faculties of the universities with which those schools are associated. But Mr. Kinzer's paper makes it very clear that there is a potential for real conflict. I happen to believe that that's true. It's a conflict that I don't think needs to occur. It's one that we should all strive to avoid.

There are going to be changes in physician behavior and physician practice. There must be accompanying changes in patient behavior and, at the same time, there must be changes in hospital administration behavior. One of those changes already under way ensures that doctors participate on boards of trustees of hospitals and, to that extent, in hospital management.

Mr. Kinzer's war pilot analogy is excellent. The language we physicians speak about the things that drive physicians today is much the same as the pilots spoke in World War II. Yet he makes one statement that I don't agree with: he says it's either total cooperation or total war; you can't come down in the middle. I don't agree with that. I think we can come down in the middle. I think we'd better come down either on the side of total cooperation or somewhere in the middle, or we will have total war.

Discussion

DR. WILBUR: I second the thoughts of many about what an excellent analogy and stimulating paper Mr. Kinzer's is, but I also have a concern along the lines that Dr. Sammons spoke of last. He makes the point that if a physician wishes to work in a freestanding operation, he or she could be excluded from the hospital staff. I think that's an artificial distinction. In one moment we are speaking of trying to get the hospital management and boards of directors together with the medical staff and in the next we are splitting into two types of physicians: those who are inside the circled wagons and those who are outside, who are regarded in Mr. Kinzer's analogy as privateers.

I think the patient should be admitted to the institution that best suits the patient's needs, and that may be a freestanding surgicenter if there is not a need for hospitalization. The fact that the physician can admit to an operating room, a surgicenter, or whatever is best and most cost effective for the patient is extremely important. In Europe, that's often not the case, and there is a sharp distinction between the hospital-based physicians and those who do not have admitting privileges. In general, there is very little quality control of the nonhospital physician.

In this country, hospital privileges and the supervision of hospital work constitute one of our best systems of ongoing hospital control. I would be very concerned if, with the growing supply of physicians, we reverted to a system in which the elite have hospital privileges and all the rest are kept on the outside.

DR. DAVID J. OTTENSMEYER: I would like to point out the danger of carrying this analogy too far.

I was an Air Force pilot in the Korean War and I assure you the first time they let me fly the plane myself, I felt I was a power unto myself. And I had an interesting follow-up experience recently. At Christmas I had the opportunity to sit down with a young man who had just graduated from Air Force flight school. I discovered that the military pilot today does not feel that he is an instrument separate either from the command structure or from the overall process that goes on in the fielding of either a land air force type of operation or a naval air force type of operation. He emphasized to me that the pilot doesn't operate separately from the control and command structure. Whereas we on a crew in the Korean War ate, lived, and drank together, they don't today. They emphasize individual crew performance, and the success or failure of a military crew is enormously dependent upon a very complex set of logistics and intelligence to put it into the field. It really has to be that way if you think about it. They are flying enormously expensive machinery. They are delivering weapons that have huge amounts of destructive power, much different from the firecrackers that we were used to twenty years ago.

I think if you want to carry the analogy into the reality of what we're dealing with today, you'll look at the airlines. The airline captain has a certain set of licensed privileges and prerogatives. Sometimes he has to make critical life-and-death decisions, but he doesn't decide when the airplane flies, where it's going to go, or what will be the purpose of the mission. He is part of a very complex organization that is designed to accomplish air transportation. I think the romantic idea of the physician sallying forth to do battle with disease is going to have to be put into perspective much more realistically. Today's physician is working in an organization that is very big, very expensive, and very dangerous, and it has to be very carefully planned.

MR. MICHAEL BROMBERG: Professor Stevens made the point earlier that maybe there never was a partnership, and I think there's some merit to that. I think society is sending us the message that there must be a partnership. I think this is what Dr. Sammons is saying, that this is something we'd better listen to. Mr. McMahon made the point that hospitals are different from carriers because hospitals have to define their mission. I think that's changing. Society is defining its mission for us, and a lot of hospitals and a lot of physicians don't like it. Some of the paranoia and fear of the unknown has arisen because of society telling hospitals to change their mission, to become partners with their doctors, to change their behavior and that of physicians.

The point that Mr. Kinzer makes that's going to come back to haunt us is the ethical consideration. I remember the time when it was considered unethical for physicians to own hospitals; then, I remember the time when the state of New York decided to protect quality by having only physicians own hospitals because if anyone else owned them quality might be sacrificed. Then New York changed that law halfway and said the owner of the hospital didn't have to be a doctor. I think that physician-managers are going to be very important. Physicians are going to have to become more involved in management. I think Mr. Kinzer's comments are going to come around full circle again.

DR. MERLIN K. DUVAL: I would like to suggest that there may be some merit in looking at this issue from a different perspective. Today in the United States is a time of enormous excesses on the supply side. We have an excess of beds. We have excess of capacity in the system. We have too many practitioners. We have too many health personnel. It's a time of unbundling too many choices, too many entry points.

Today is also, however, a time of restraint on the financial resources, especially in view of the phenomenon of budget neutrality. That adds up, in my judgment, to a very bad situation. It means that there have to be some very important failures as well as some important successes. If this is true, in the context of fighting for a piece of the action in the face of budget neutrality, I would ask if partnerships could be coequal. I wonder whether or not that which drives the machine in this nation is such as to drive us toward an unequal partnership. A test case if you wish, but if physicians' fees by 1986 are in fact incorporated in DRGs, to whom are we to give the money?

DR. HARVEY ESTES: Mr. Kinzer's air crew was there because somebody wanted it to be there and wanted it enough to pay for it. They wanted it so badly that they were willing to pay for building the ships and deploying them in that location. I think we've been in that position as an industry in the past. The public wanted it so badly they were willing to pay anything for it, but now that's eroded and we're at a point where we can no longer count on that support. It's more like the situation in the Vietnam War—we're there without support and without a willingness to pay. That's another part of the analogy that I think we ought to take a look at.

DR. JOSEPH F. BOYLE: Perhaps the most challenging thrust I've heard this morning was given by Dr. Wallace. Perhaps we have the answer to the wrong question. Of if we don't have the answer, we are certainly looking for the answer to the wrong question. When I first went into practice, there was an unlimited opportunity for hospitals and physicians working together to effect the greatest good in the area of taking care of patients. At the same time, both physicians and hospitals could not help but prosper. There was also real conflict between the interests of the people who were running the hospitals and the interests of the doctors. The director of the hospital council of Southern California once told me that clearly we were not in the same business—I was in the doctor business and he was in the hospital business.

In the interim from then until now, there has been such a change in the environment that perhaps we have not developed the feedback system that would tell us how we have changed our own internal organization in order to respond. We are at a point where there is not only a new level of accountability, but there are also new opportunities. The time when physicians can ignore the consequences of their own actions is long past. Hospitals may still have the option to ignore what happens to doctors, but that's one of the facts of life!

Perhaps we can begin to develop the sensors that will allow us to take some of the oscillations out of the system. At the same time I think we have to very clearly define our mission. Our mission has been to provide excellence in patient care. If we approach this from the standpoint that we all are accountable, that there are other players in the game than just doctors and hospitals, perhaps we can reach that point a little bit sooner.

PROFESSOR THOMPSON: The question is not whether there's going to be total independence of physicians. The question is in the area of the constraints and who sets them. Physicians have accepted a lot of constraints having to do with quality. Are they going to accept constraints on costs? It's extremely important for physicians to become involved in setting these constraints. The time when the hospital supplies the goods to enable the physician to treat the patients however he wants to is gone. Anyone who has looked at the DRG data, particularly the cost data, at the wide variation within one DRG that you reduce by keying in the physician will realize this has nothing to do with the severity of illness.

ness. It has to do with physicians' patterns of practice. We just can't afford this kind of wide variation.

PROFESSOR STEVENS: I hope we're going to see physicians who are very anxious but realize they must be attuned to what's going on. I worry about that.

The point I really want to make is, who is the hospital? When we talk about hospitals, which groups of people represent hospitals? We're talking very little about boards of trustees. You could argue that CEOs and physicians involved in hospital medical staffs are likely to be very much more informed than boards of trustees of voluntary hospitals. I hope at some point in the discussion we come back to what expertise we expect from boards of trustees.

DR. SAMMONS: I agree with Dr. Thompson that practice patterns are going to change. The difference is whether they occur because the state of the art and the concern for quality says change is appropriate or whether they occur because the screws are being tightened on a financial base in an institutional setting that says to the physician, "You will change or you will go!"

The hospital must preserve the integrity and the ethics of the practice regardless of cost, and I think that's what most doctors in the country believe. I think that's the way most of us have always practiced: the first thing we worry about is the patient; we worry about the costs later. Unfortunately, the forces at work today are going to keep much of that from happening in the future. It really doesn't matter whether you're talking about proprietary hospitals or not-for-profit hospitals. The same thing is going to happen to both of them. Money is in short supply. All third party payers are reducing the level of payment.

One wonders whether at the end of the year we will have a happy medical staff that has been treating the same sort of people they've always treated, or whether we will have a group of the unhappiest people in the world who will feel that they can no longer practice good quality medicine.

I am convinced that we are going to see more closed staffs in hospitals in the next three to five years than anybody dreams or than we've ever seen. Every lawyer in the country will be increasing his standard of living substantially as a result of the lawsuits that will follow. It's not just going to be the hospitals that decide to do it; the doctors themselves will be deciding to do it. Soon the medical staff of an institution will go to the administration and say, "We want to put together a PPO and we want you to help us. You bring in the management expertise because we're concerned about our practice load." It's not a very big step from there to saying to the administration, "Let's protect the practice even more; let's close the staff. We don't need all of these ob-gyn men running around loose, the birth rate's down. We don't need all these cardiologists running around loose." Take any specialty you want. That little step is going to change the historic relationships between physicians and patients and between physicians and hospitals in this country as much as technology has changed them, as much as the proprietary investor-owned system has changed them, as much as the DRG payment mechanism is going to change them.

If you look at the people who are beginning to worry about the ability to practice quality medicine, they cut across all lines. Unless doctors and hospitals can sit down and explain to each other what their problems are, they will never resolve them. I don't think anybody has to worry about the DRG payment mechanism in the next five years because it has so many pass-throughs built into it that you can steal the system blind if you really want to. You're not going to upset labor in the hospital because you're just going to pass that on through to the government. You're not going to upset the teaching hospitals a great deal because you're going to have a complicated formula that gets worse every year that passes through the costs of education in some fashion. They're going to keep changing the Medicare payment mechanisms until all the old people either get tired of it and tell them to stop or find a way to beat the system to continue to take care of them.

Four years or five years from now is when the screw really gets tightened, and we're going to see all of the fallout. There must be a clear understanding on the part of the management of the hospital as to what physicians need in order to effectively treat their patients. And we must have doctors who are better educated and more attuned to the financial resources of the institution and how they can be managed. If we don't have both, then all of the other things that we are worried about are going to pale by comparison, because it is the quality of health care that is at risk in this country today. It is not the financial stability of the federal government.

PROFESSOR GINZBERG: If you have more doctors coming into the system than the system really needs, and if you have more beds than the system really is using now, and if you're going to have a lot of new facilities, and if you're going to have just the same amount of money, it's inevitable that the quality will get worse and worse in this system. What you have is a disproportion between the amount of resources you need for quality and the amount of resources that have to be fed by the limited money. There is no way of achieving the balance between quality and resources unless you face up to some serious issues.

The existing institutions—the hospitals on the one side and the physicians on the other—are on what I would call a microlevel. They cannot solve this one. It is not solvable in those terms. They can get together a little bit better or a little bit worse, but the question is really a systemwide problem now: you have more people trying to make a living from a definable amount of money, and that will inevitably reduce your quality.

We always had "dollar control" over quality. It was very simple. The voluntary boards of the big hospitals had to meet some kind of a budget and we permitted just so much deficit, and that was all the money that the doctors had to work with. Within those budgets, we took care of whatever the hospital could provide. A lot of doctors wanted to buy more for their patients but couldn't. A lot of patients were not well taken care of at all; we didn't pay attention to them. In the last twenty-five years, though, we've been on a fantastic spree. We defined quality by saying that you could use all the money you like forever. That is an impossible system. It doesn't work. Now we are going to be pushed back and forced to come up with some kind of budgetary constraint on the system again.

The situation is complicated by the fact that we decided along the way that all Americans were entitled to quality. I don't think we ever believed it, but we said it. Therefore, we have some real tough problems that go way beyond doctor-hospital partnership.

DR. EDGAR DAVIS: I think those who control the resources will ultimately have to address the question just raised by Dr. Ginzberg which is, what is an appropriate budget limit? What are appropriate expenditures for a firm in its employee benefit program? What represents appropriate public expenditures?

If some structural process isn't found by which hospitals, physicians, and those groups of, say, businesses, find a way to exchange an understanding of this system, its needs, and its dilemmas, then there will be very shortsighted, harsh, insensitive, budget-oriented procedures made by those controlling the resources, particularly within the private sector. Anyone with a budget in a firm that is attempting to control expenditures and maximize revenues is always going to favor lower unit costs, lower premium costs, etc., and we will face the dilemma of needing to understand at what point we have achieved a level of desired efficiency in the system and at what level we are beginning to harm the system. I don't know how we're going to know that unless we have a fuller role in the partnership on which this conference is based.

DR. JOHN E. AFFELDT: The concept has been put forth here, and quite properly I believe, that boards of trustees will clearly have to take a more active role and responsibility than they have in the past. Professor Stevens properly asked the question, are they capable of that?

I'm aware that trustees are forming organizations, just as administrators have organizations of administrators and physicians have organizations of physicians. Some of those trustee organizations are approaching the JCAH and asking for help. They are, in effect, asking if the JCAH will look at this and consider the possibility of setting up some mechanism for evaluating boards of trustees. I'm not in a position to predict whether the JCAH will or will not do that, but I do find it interesting that that voice is coming from organized trustees.

MR. MCMAHON: For some twenty years we had annual increases in hospital costs. They averaged between 15 and 18 percent per year at times when the gross national product was growing at 5 to 9 percent. As Professor Ginzberg said, that can't continue because, if it does, we will have a totally unacceptable level of expenditure of GNP, enough to threaten all other kinds of things including the automobile industry, the airline industry, the travel industry, food, shelter, clothing, and public services.

We haven't been asked to stop that increase altogether. We've been asked to lower it to somewhere in the 8 or 9 percent range, which doesn't represent the same kind of threat. If we do that, the administrator side and the medical side can turn their attention to a kind of operation that doesn't threaten quality.

DRGS are not the cause of our problem today. They are a factor of public policy change that says, "Get those damned things down to 8 or 9 percent increase per year and if we're not going to do it this way, we're going to do it some other way!"

We are still going to experience substantial increases in the money flowing to health care services, certainly enough to protect quality, if we only change our way of doing things as some advisers would have us do. Although the incentives are different, they are still liberal enough to provide us with some money.

Now, on the matter of boards of trustees, I'm not dissatisfied with their performance. Maybe if some of them are inadequate to the task, they represent an institution unable to define its mission that might pass quietly from the scene.

I think letting the marketplace work its will, letting those institutions find ways to govern themselves, to define their missions, to bring about harmony and constructive tension within the institution is probably the best way to do it. If we get a governmental solution, even a joint commission, I think we're likely to make some huge mistakes.

Frankly, we have too many businessmen and socially conscious women making up some of these trustee organizations, instead of the real leaders the board needs who are likely to be busy back home doing other kinds of things.

DR. NELSON: We've been examining the relationship between the medical staff, hospital administration, and hospital board in a sort of macrofashion. I'd like to take advantage of a new perspective from the viewpoint of a medical staff member, which obviously will be biased and probably simplistic.

The first thing I'd like to question is the role of the board. The board of trustees of a hospital gets together every couple of months, has dinner, and goes about its business, the most important feature of which is to hire a CEO. The reason that's so important is because in day-to-day trusteeship, the board is at the mercy of the information given to them by the CEO.

The second thing that the board does is promote expansion of the facility and raise money for that expansion. Nobody salutes the board member for making a smaller facility. While the board has "fiduciary responsibility" and "quality responsibility," it only rarely exerts those other than by being a watchdog. To do so would invite conflict, and publicity about the conflict is almost never good. Insofar as the board is concerned, it is virtually never in their best interest to raise a fuss.

Hospital management runs the hospital and keeps the books, hires enough people to make sure the boilerplate is in place when the JCAH people come around. Management wants a happy board and a happy medical staff, so it's virtually never in their best interest to raise a fuss.

If I have an argument with Mr. Kinzer's analogy of wartime pilots and present-day doctors, it would be the portrayal of physicians as combatants. Physicians want a hassle-free environment in which to do their business. They don't want to make a fuss. If a physician has to make a fuss, he usually goes past the CEO and the board, directly to the public, and then in a standoff he usually doesn't lose.

So one of our problems is that these corrections in hospital cybernetics have to be triggered externally, since none of the three legs wants to make a fuss. The kinds of corrections we've talked about—the availability of money, irresistible public opinion, and mandated certificate of need—will almost certainly involve larger fluctuations than would be desirable. The stress that will come with those kinds of fluctuations is going to be painful. Almost certainly, at some time down the stream, the American public isn't going to take easily to rationing. I think there will be a reaction that will make the first swing in the feedback loop look modest. When the reaction in the corrections occurs one decade from now it may be tremendous.

PROFESSOR REINHARDT: I've always been puzzled by what mandates physicians think they have in connection with quality. Where on that quality versus cost curve do physicians believe the public wants them to be? Is it always at that point of maximum technically feasible quality regardless of how much it costs?

The DRG mechanism has been accused of reducing the quality of care. An economist would say, "Yes, it might," and that's an issue we might discuss: how much money is a little change in quality actually worth? And, we might even be more concrete and say, "Don't just tell me quality goes down, but tell me exactly what it is that would go down," because what you might view as quality I, as a taxpayer or a patient, might not consider as quality.

I think we must be very specific about quality. What exactly is it that must go when we constrain resources or when we input a different pricing mechanism? Second, do physicians really and sincerely believe that they have a mandate from the public to deliver the maximum technically feasible quality regardless of how much that costs? Or, do they think it legitimate to discuss where on that curve a society should be?

I think the taxpayers have the right to decide how much quality they wish to buy through the public sector. It would not be at all outrageous to suggest, as in the Grace Commission report, that the government has a certain level of quality that it will buy for people and no more. I don't think it's a crime to talk that way. I think that should be more openly discussed. The real problem comes if we say that a certain amount of health care is all we want to buy for the publicly financed patient; should we then allow private wealthy patients to buy more quality? Do we allow different Americans to be at different points on that curve?

That is the real vexing problem of this decade. If we want that feedback loop, and we shall within the next decade, it might trigger a populace reaction that might ultimately lead to socialized medicine in this country. If we are too far spread on that curve, it's conceivable that those are the real dangers, not so much that we will give up some quality. The real problem is exactly whose quality is it that we're going to give up.

Mr. McMahon mentioned that we can't go on spending as much as we do on health care. Actually we really could keep running at the present pace for a number of decades. If we continue to the year 2000 having an annual increase in health care expenditure of 15 percent while the GNP grows only at 9 percent, then in the year 2000 one-third of the GNP will go to health care. But this will not bankrupt us, remarkably because the nonhealth GNP per capita would still be higher than it is today, so we could still have everything we have now, plus a little extra. It is, in fact, economically feasible to keep spending the way we do. There's no macroeconomic imperative that would make us spend less.

MR. SHELTON: The private sector is already beginning to try to put budget constraints on health care programs. For some time now they've been very active in encouraging the development and growth of HMOs and other forms of alternative delivery systems as well as benefit programs that encourage outpatient care and so forth.

We're in the process of developing programs to identify the high cost provider who is out of synch with his associates in order to either educate him and bring him in line or exclude him from the program. But there's something else developing that is going to put intense pressure on the relationship between hospitals and physicians. These are the limited access capitated plans. Unlike PPOS, these programs are mandatory. They do not allow the individual to go outside the provider panel for services. The provider panel is generally selected based on cost although, of course, there are quality considerations as well. I would say that there are things developing other than DRGS that are going to have a very significant impact on the relationship between physicians and hospitals.

MR. MCNERNEY: I've heard the administrator described today as someone who's concerned with the happiness index, keeping the hotel going, maximizing the minimum trouble. I heard the board characterized as a semibenign group of people who are awakening, but only very slowly. And the medical staff is anxiously milling around, wondering exactly how to relate to management and to governance.

That is not the world I see. First of all, the amount of vertical and horizontal integration in this country is literally revolutionary among hospitals, and a lot of the leadership comes from the hospital administrator.

We're talking about institutions that are doing well. They are not only getting into upfront ambulatory care, skilled nursing home care, and hospice care; they are also joining with other institutions and forming holding companies, and those holding companies are forming wholly owned subsidiaries that are getting into a variety of profit-producing ventures that help to provide the capital to make all this innovation necessary.

At the head of such hospitals is a strong executive responding to a new set of forces. For the sake of our discussion we must begin to think of those types of individuals because they are there. Some of them, to be sure, are remote from the patient as these horizontal systems grow.

Boards are not as passive as they used to be either. In fact, if you just look at the turnover of administrators in this country, which is large, you can see that boards are a lot more businesslike than you might have seen about five or ten years ago. Also, they're highly supportive of these new ventures and much tougher about the budget without apology.

As far as the medical staff is concerned, we have a lot more full-time medical directors, a lot more part-time department heads, a lot more M.D.s on the governing structure. This is not being debated; it's going on!

Our discussion would be a lot more to the point if it were focused on what is going on now, let alone what will probably be coming.

DR. COOPER: The problem of how many physicians we need in this country is purely legal. The important question is, how much care and what kind of care are we willing to provide the people in this country? From the answer comes the number of physicians that we need. One can say that we're going to have an older population or we have new technology and therefore we ought to have more physicians. If you're going to take money out of the system and reduce the amount of support for medical care, it's going to reduce the need for physicians.

I would also like to point out one thing: U.S. medical schools are no longer keepers of the gate on how many physicians there are in this country. We have 127 medical schools in this country. We have more than doubled the number of entering students, and that has been reflected in the output in the past decade and a half. However, over the last two years the number of entering medical school students has fallen for the first time since about the thirties, after the reduction in the number of medical schools following the Flexner report.

So, the medical student population has decreased two years in a row and our projections are for it to decrease again in 1984. There is, then, a feedback loop. It's a bad one and it's sluggish, but the number of applicants is going down. Even though the feedback loop is sluggish, the response in terms of the number of physicians is probably better than any predictors can make of the number of physicians we need.

We have at least 10,000 American students going to medical schools outside the United States. The number of U.S. graduates of foreign medical schools applying for first-year positions through the residency matching plan is going up and up. We now have more than 2,500, and the number is more than doubling every year. Also, the number of alien foreign medical graduates applying for first-year positions is rising very sharply.

Professor Reinhardt asked, What do the people want in medical care? How much quality? I'd like to ask if he thinks there's a difference between what individuals think about their own medical care and what they think about the quality of medical care generally. The polls have shown that patients still think their doctor is in the highest ranked profession, but when they are asked about medical care in the abstract, they don't have such high opinions of it.

I think those two points are important because that's where the physician and hospital are going to enter into a kind of conflict, not only between themselves but also with the federal government and other payers or with patients themselves about the quality of care.

PROFESSOR REINHARDT: I think people are essentially of two minds. They wish to purchase for their fellow citizens a certain level of care, probably somewhat lower than the quality they wish to purchase for themselves. I think the system has responded to these desires with an increasing commercialization of the health care system, and that is a natural response to this attitude.

We have the same attitude in this country toward education. We have no trouble at all with an educational system that delivers one quality of care to some folks, but we must have the best for our own children. This country tolerates that, and, in fact, almost encourages the tradition. We do it with bread, we do it with wine, and we do it with basic services like education.

This is probably also the American ethos in health care. I've come to that conclusion after watching this debate for a decade. The logical conclusion of everything I've ever heard, here or elsewhere, is that this is a two-tier nation for everything. It is unrealistic to assume that that wouldn't also apply in health care.

So, the issue before us as far as public policy is concerned is what should the quality of that bottom tier be like?

DR. DAVID E. ROGERS: One of the things that troubles me greatly, particularly when we begin to have a dollar squeeze, is that we in medicine have virtually no way of measuring quality. You and I might agree that a certain doctor practices quality of care, but to translate that to a congressman is very, very difficult.

I am afraid that with the big cost constraints we will do some very destructive things to quality. We don't have any good yardsticks to use within medicine and that's the rock on which we are now foundering. We talk about "quality of care," and I think I know it when I see it, but I have a terrible time explaining it to a nonphysician group.

MR. JOHN IGLEHART: I think it's important to underscore the great contradictions among politicians. While they pursue cost containment on the one hand, they also pursue with equal vigor the "Baby Doe" phenomenon and organ transplantation legislation. I would decry their unwillingness to admit the contradiction, to recognize it, and to try to deal with it.

MR. JOHN W. COLLOTON: I have some difficulty with the pessimism that Mr. Kinzer has with respect to the willingness of individual physicians to examine their practice patterns in the context of the new economic reality. I would like to focus for a moment on a microlevel of what one sees now at the institutional operating level.

Every place I look, I see physicians and professional organizations like the AAMC and the AHA and the specialty societies coming to grips with these realities through a broad series of educational programs and organizational initiatives at the individual hospital level. They display a remarkable willingness to review and amend practice styles to assure quality patient care.

In our institutions, I work with a thousand and fifty physicians every day who are very willing to take on the DRG-related questions of unproductive practice patterns. In fact, they're more eager to get into it than the hospital administration. They are coming to us for all of the comparative data, right down the individual DRG and the individual physician practice pattern within their particular specialty. I think they are doing this because they see the destiny of their respective departments tied to the destiny of the university hospital.

If we want to be objective about it, I think we will agree that there are lots of economic shortcomings in hospital operations. If you look at the sixty-four university-owned teaching hospitals in this country, you see staff-to-occupied-bed ratios ranging from nine down to four staff per occupied bed. You see general expense—that is, nonsalaried expenditure—ranging from $254,000 per bed down to $35,000 per bed. You see studies from Harvard showing that in some teaching hospitals 47 percent of the laboratory work is unrelated to patient outcome.

Under the new incentives, the good hospital directors are not attempting to manage medical care. They're attempting to stimulate the staff to look at medical practice in the context of economics. They're attempting to provide the supporting services to make that possible.

I'm not nearly as pessimistic as Mr. Kinzer about the willingness of individual physicians and groups of physicians to do that.

If the hospital of the future is well managed and efficient and directs itself to quality patient care, recognizing that there is some $300 billion and an awful lot of opportunity out there, we ought to be more optimistic about being able to succeed in a collaborative context.

PROFESSOR PATRICIA DANZON: I would like to return to the question of the schizophrenia of the public toward how much we should spend on health care. It's not just a question of how much we want to spend on the poor versus how much we want to spend on ourselves. The real dilemma is how much we want to spend on ourselves when we're sick versus how much we want to spend when we're well. When we're sick, we're paying with insurance dollars; we have paid the premium, so now we're only paying the copayment portion, not the full cost. When we're well and we're paying the insurance premium, we are paying the full cost. This distinction creates what insurance economists call moral hazard: that is, once you've got the insurance, you tend to want to spend more than you would before you had the insurance.

It's this problem of moral hazard that leads to a lot of the tension between how much physicians want to spend because they're catering to the patients who are sick—who are not paying the cost at that point—and how much politicians want to spend when they are setting the budgets and have to pay the full insurance premiums.

That problem of moral hazard is one reason why we would not want to leave cost containment decisions to individual physicians, but rather have some constraints set by hospitals, because the physician is exposed to the patient at a point where the patient is not paying the full cost.

PROFESSOR CLARK HAVIGHURST: I want to return to some earlier questions about the nature of the doctor-hospital relationship. David Kinzer stated his preference for physician involvement as opposed to actual hospital control over management of doctors. I think that needs to be viewed as a statement of an ideal.

I think Dr. Ottensmeyer's point about how commercial airlines operate as opposed to how aircraft carriers operate is very interesting. It suggests that Mr. Kinzer's idea is essentially a romantic one, though one that has served us very well and should continue to be held as an ideal. In other words, many hospitals could be run using the old model in which physicians are involved in management, and act responsibly in that capacity, but aren't controlled in any sense by the hospital itself. But that isn't necessarily the universal model. Indeed, I don't think it would be appropriate for all hospitals to do business in that way. Different management philosophies and techniques will work in different situations. Depending on the kinds of physicians involved, one technique may be useful in one setting and not in another. For example, if the physician staff is all trained in the Caribbean, there might be a little reluctance to accord them total independence. For different population groups you may find that different arrangements within hospitals may be more or less acceptable. Some hospitals may find that their particular circumstances call for controlling some doctors and not others.

So, while I respect the statement of the ideal, I would like to make a plea for maintaining flexibility in order that hospitals may better deal with the particular circumstances in which they find themselves. In other words, we should not think that there is only one right way of organizing a hospital to deliver services. There should be freedom for various approaches, and all hospitals should have competitive incentives to attract good physicians. Most of the best physicians will aspire to practice in settings where their independence is maintained, so hospitals are under pressure to accord independence to physicians who are capable of exercising it.

Hospitals also have to attract patients and they have to attract good doctors who will attract patients. They have to provide satisfactory settings in which the doctors and patients are generally content. It seems to me that this marketplace may, in fact, help us to find the best ways of organizing for the mission of patient care in every hospital. We don't want to be talking about designing an ideal system. We want to be talking about having a system in which each institution will strive to do the best it can with the resources at its disposal.

DR. ANLYAN: I would like to ask David Ottensmeyer, in your analogy using the modern commercial pilot, you said that the pilot operates under certain constraints; how much are these the constraints of the FAA and how much of them are the constraints of airline companies? In other words, is there freedom for the individual hospital working within state standards and federal standards?

DR. OTTENSMEYER: The vast majority of the legal constraints are from the FAA and the transportation board, but certainly there's a vast range of privilege that is given to one airline or another as to what the pilot can decide and what the pilot can't decide.

You find in a small commuter airline that the individual pilot gasses up the plane and collects the tickets and so forth. This pilot has a great deal to do with the decisions that are made about any one flight. On the other hand, with American Airlines, the pilot walks in and sits down in the left seat and is given a computer printout that is his flight plan. He has very little decision-making freedom.

MR. MCMAHON: There still is an assumption that the doctor is calling the shots about the quality or extent or amount of patient care, but experience doesn't bear that out, especially when you look at changes in patient behavior with the installation of cost sharing in benefit programs.

A lot of medical care is patient-initiated, and I think we may see even more of that. I think business is proving that cost sharing does have an effect. There are going to be times when patients begin to say, "Do I really need that, Doctor?" Then there are going to be implications for the financial viability of the institution—not just from government interference on behalf of Medicare beneficiaries, but from patient involvement and patient questioning about the extent of medical care. These are going to increase both the tension and the need for cooperation.

DR. SAMMONS: One thing that I have said repeatedly over the last several years is that doctors and hospitals are inseparable. They are inseparable for all the reasons that all of us know, and we must not let them be separated because of money. So there is going to be a need for a more realistic approach on the part of all three partners—patients, doctors, and hospitals—beginning now.

I think every doctor in this country would like to believe that he or she is always operating at the vertical rise of Professor Reinhardt's cost versus quality curve. Whether or not that's true remains to be seen, but the fear is that the fallback from the vertical rise will be dictated not by considerations of patients' needs, but simply by costs, and that that is the determinant that will impair quality. Whether that's true or not, I don't know. We'll have to wait and see, but we are in a two-tier system. We've always been in one.

I have jokingly made the argument from time to time that the most overtreated people in the world are the very rich and the very poor who live near teaching hospitals. This is only half facetious; the very rich because they go out and buy medical treatment and the very poor because in the old days being near the teaching hospitals was an absolutely marvelous thing. We may find some day that all this business of a one-tier system of health care in this country was absolutely right, that what Karen Davis and Teddy Kennedy had a whole decade to improve on was nothing more than the same kind of facade that most of us said it was at the outset. I personally believe that with the DRG system we will go through the same exercise all over again.

4

Four Pathways for Hospitals and Physicians: Introduction

PAUL M. ELLWOOD, JR., M.D.

So far we have agreed that hospitals and doctors have maintained a rather unique symbiotic relationship that is apparently advantageous to both. Despite the fact that there are overwhelming arguments that inpatient care is a product of this joint relationship, the two sides, as Professors Thompson and Stevens pointed out, have managed to be amazingly independent of one another. In part, this is because of the professional status of the physician and his desire—to use Mr. Kinzer's metaphor—to continue to function as a sort of fighter pilot. Partly it flows from the perception that a significant potential exists for economic conflict of interest when physicians control or own hospitals.

But perhaps the crucial factor allowing physicians and hospitals to maintain their arm's length autonomy is the way in which medical care has been paid for in the United States. By focusing the payer's attention on the complex maze of seemingly unrelated and individual services, this payment system has obscured the underlying fact that the cost of patient care is really defined by combined actions and decisions of doctors and hospital administrators.

We at this conference have identified five or six factors that underlie a change in this relationship. The first is the advent of prospective payment where the third party puts the hospital at risk for its medical staff's behavior. Physicians have as much impact on the cost per discharge as the hospital does (or more), and cooperation is vital if they are to hit their prospective reimbursement targets. But the DRG system really passes no direct incentives on to physicians that would guarantee their cooperation, which leads to what Dr. Wallace would call "aberrant feedback" in the current state of affairs. Very few physicians are motivated to work much more closely with the hospital as a result of the introduction of DRGs.

The second factor is the oversupply of both doctors and hospital beds. This creates intense pressure and competition between physicians and between hospitals and, as Dr. Sammons pointed out, between hospitals and physicians. It has contributed to significant anxiety on the part of doctors and has led them to join any variety of organizations that promised to deliver them patients.

We have two health plans in a community that are competing with each other. One has 2,300 doctors and one has 230 doctors. Both have been successful. Each has enrolled in the health plan about 160,000 people. The one that has 230 doctors in it has delivered ten times as many patients per doctor as the other, and this shows up in their behavior. Only 5 percent of the physicians in the plan with 230 physicians have chosen to join other health plans, whereas more than 50 percent of the physicians in the health plan that has 2,300 doctors in it have chosen to join other organizations.

The third phenomenon is the cost consciousness that third-party payers, government, industry, and health insurers, have assumed in seeking respite from escalating health care costs. Third-party payers are becoming aware that the crisis in fees and charges is really not the important measure of costs. They are seeking reimbursement savings from reduced utilization of health care. Every place we go in the country now, talking to business roundtables, they admit that what they are really concerned about is the number of days that their work force spends in a hospital. One of the kinds of behaviors that we're starting to see from third parties now is limiting provider choice. This is not confined to Medicaid. Blue Cross of Kansas City now has a plan in which consumers can obtain the usual set of health benefits—not an extraordinary set of health benefits—only by going to a selected set of doctors and hospitals. Hewlett-Packard in Silicone Valley has begun doing everything it can to encourage its employees to limit their choices and go to a single institution, El Camino Hospital.

The fourth phenomenon is the industrialization of health care, which is both supporting and feeding off this competitive revolution. Organized, managed health care systems that can efficiently produce quality care seem to be thriving in this new environment. Cost competitiveness allows them to take advantage of efficiencies that were never before possible. For example, U.S. Health Care is one of the new proprietary national medical care firms. They pay primary physicians a certain amount per capita to purchase health services on behalf of their patients, and they've found that it works very well. They don't have to take a lot of risks; they can have the physicians take the risks. They can play off the natural competitiveness that exists within the health system by saying to the primary physicians, "We'll let you buy the surgeon's or superspecialist's services. You're in charge." This turns out to be an inexpensive way to get into the business, and it is the kind of idea that national firms grab onto when they see any inkling that it works.

The fifth phenomenon is the vertical integration of services by providers, which is really the primary thrust of the new health care corporations. They are placing insurance, marketing, professional medical services, hospital services, and extended care under common management and, by doing this, they can much more aggressively market and balance their resources.

Much has been made of the notion that one should select cost-effective hospitals and doctors under these new rules of medical care, but these national, vertically integrated firms have found it equally important to balance the numbers and types of beds and hospitals and drugs and so forth with the needs of their patient population. They don't want any extra mouths to feed. To my way of thinking, this phenomenon would tend to exaggerate perhaps more than anything the oversupply of physicians and hospital beds that may exist in the country.

Finally, the sixth phenomenon is the hospital-physician interdependence that replaces independence and autonomy. Patient flows and volumes are no longer a function of the ability of an individual physician to go out and be successful as a practitioner and refer patients into the hospital. The price of an individual encounter with a doctor or a day in the hospital is no longer the real basis for measuring the cost effectiveness of the health system. Rather, price competition occurs at the level of provider systems, such as Blue Cross, or providers that are organized in HMOs or PPOs. Doctors and hospitals in competitive positions are no longer defined by their practice patterns or their costs but by the company they keep.

Take, for example, Stanford Hospital, where two groups of practitioners practice: the faculty of the medical school and a large multispecialty group practice. The behavior of both these groups determines what the bottom line is for that hospital, not one or the other segment. The effect of this has been to change the minimum size of an efficient medical care firm. It used to be that a medical care firm really only had to be large enough to wash out actuarial risk; it could be fifty doctors and 50,000 enrollments. But with DRGs, the whole hospital as an institution and its entire medical staff become the risk group and so the minimum size firm becomes a group of perhaps two hundred doctors using a four-hundred bed hospital. Now, all these factors have pushed the existing system toward organized, proactive, competitive units that are vertically integrated. So that, in summary, physicians can now destroy a hospital's financial position in a prospectively paid system, whatever the cost structure of the hospital. At the same time, an affiliation with an expensive hospital can limit a physician's patient base and undermine his practice.

There are four basic pathways that are being speculated about as hospitals and doctors try to cope with these six phenomena. All four are represented at our conference today. One speaker, Dr. David Ottensmeyer, is a physician who manages a hospital. The second, Mr. Stanley Nelson, is a hospital administrator who manages a set of physicians in a very large group practice. The third, Dr. Joseph F. Boyle, is a physician who feels that in this interchange between doctors and hospitals the physicians have to organize themselves much better to have an organization that's parallel to that of the hospitals so that they can function as equals in the environment. And, finally, I will be talking about cooperative arrangements.

1984 and Beyond: Physicians and Hospitals in a New Era

DAVID J. OTTENSMEYER, M.D.

As can be seen from your agenda, the subject matter of this paper about physicians and hospitals in a new era refers to the hospital organizational model in which the physician owns and operates the institution. To define terms, I intend to talk about a model with physician management and control. I do not believe that ownership is relevant one way or the other, although such would assure at least control by governance. To me, the central issues are, who sets the agenda for the institution? and what are the risks and commitments necessary from all constituencies in the institution relative to that agenda?

I have reviewed the historical and worldwide relationship of the medical profession to hospitals and health care organizations. I have also examined the posture of the medical profession and the hospital industry one to another based upon realities of the relationship and deeply held values on the part of both. I conclude that the basis for the extreme tensions that now exist within the great partnership is society's health care agenda, which is tearing apart the partnership. I suggest that the response to society's health care agenda by hospitals will be driven by organizational issues, including the need for strong, centralized management; marketing; efficient resource allocation; improved productivity; and diversification. I conclude that the interests of the organization and the medical profession are historically and generally inconsistent.

Thus, we arrive at the crossroads and are in a quest for a new model. The existing model, or status quo, seems to be dysfunctional because it is a fragmented and decentralized system poorly adapted to evaluating risks, establishing goals, and allocating resources. It is one devoted to past values and it remains dominated by professional decision making, which is heavily oriented to the agenda of the medical profession rather than that of the organization or the health care consumer.

In place of the status quo, there seems now to be emerging what, for lack of a better term, has been called "the corporate model." It is the organizational response to the demand for change. It is characterized by centralization and much stronger management control. Concentration of capital and innovative financing of both revenues and capital needs are important objectives. Management information systems constitute its sensory system. Productivity improvement is considered the key to survival in an environment of declining resources. The market orientation is an increasing concern of the medical corporation with emphasis upon service acceptability, access convenience, and pricing. There is a distinct subordination of the role of the medical profession in institutional decision making.

All of this is creating an intense clash of values. The realities of corporate medicine just listed, plain and simply, undermine the authority of the medical profession, authority that the profession has worked so hard to maintain for a hundred years. It impairs the profession's independence, most particularly independence of the health care organization, and, as a result, strengthens the organization or hospital. It enhances the stature of management in the health care organization, a process that has never been viewed with favor by the medical profession. The trade-off appears to be a corresponding impairment of the medical profession's influence and role in the institution. It weakens the dependency of society on the medical profession. Certainly, as the focus of health care consumers is shifted toward major corporate medical competitors, this is a troublesome challenge to some of the most sacred tenets of the profession relative to their role in the health care process and the doctor-patient relationship.

The marketing orientation previously mentioned elevates the status of consumers by changing them from patients to customers—customers who want to be informed, who want to be prospectively involved in decisions, who want to include the issue of price in the exchange, and who no longer accept that "the doctor knows best." Inevitably, as the consumer gains such authority, it is that much authority of which the provider is deprived. These changes have altered and will alter the rules of medical competition. Whereas the medical profession has been so successful in controlling the behavior of its membership with the doctrine of professionalism, codes of medical ethics, systems of licensure, and influence (if not control) over access to the profession, now these normative influences are rapidly crumbling away. From the current code of ethics of the American Medical Association, references to competitive behavior among physicians have been almost totally expunged. The clash of values is no better seen than in the "turf" battles now erupting between the medical profession on one hand and the health care organizations on the other—organizations interested in diversification of their business and provision of the health care services that their marketing studies show to be of interest to consumers, in direct competition with physicians.

If the situation is as I have described and the tensions are as I have depicted, I would like to turn to a possible response for the medical profession, and I would hasten to say that I am speaking now very much as a physician, a member of the medical profession, and as a hospital administrator whose institution has to prosper with a hospital whose medical staff is totally integrated into the fabric of the hospital.

I believe that the hour is late and I am concerned that the medical profession is not formulating a response that deals with reality. I see the logical representative of the profession, the American Medical Association, spending enormous time, energy, and attention on the "formulation of a health care agenda for the American people." To me this somehow fails to recognize that the agenda will be, and very probably already has been, established by society and its representative decision makers in the Congress. With remarkable unanimity of purpose, they have moved over the last two years to codify that objective into economic reality.

To me the response of the medical profession should be a commitment to the organizational solution. Moreover, I think that it is in the best interests of the medical profession and, parenthetically, I believe it will be in the best interests of health care organizations as competitive units, if the medical profession will recognize the opportunity and will move to co-opt the organization—a move to retain its authority, its influence, and its prime role in American medicine, recognizing that the "action" is going to be in health care corporations. The central maneuver in this scenario should be the establishment of the hospital-based medical staff, a staff committed to the success of that institution and one that accepts the risks of the institution as the risks of the medical staff. The hospital medical staff can move into such a relationship by employment, by contract, or by joint venture. The relationship I propose is a very extensive bonding quite unlike the voluntary self-governing medical staff we have known heretofore.

Group practices, which constitute the prototype physician organization in the medical profession, constitute a distinct and highly workable vehicle for joint venture undertakings with health care organizations, especially hospitals. The MeSH organization that Dr. Ellwood will discuss later is an example. Physician ownership is an obvious course, but an unlikely one considering the undercapitalization of the medical profession. Finally, the key mechanism to movement of the medical profession into the health care organization is the incorporation of physician managers at middle and upper levels of management in hospitals. There they can convince and assure the medical profession that its goals, interests, and values are heard, understood, and incorporated into the organization's agenda.

I submit to you that physician executives are logical and desirable as chief executive officers of medical corporations of the future as these hospitals move to build a new relationship with physicians.

Is this approach of the physician-centered medical corporation rational? I believe that it is, because it serves the corporation well and can resolve the intense clash of values now disturbing the whole system. It has the promise of creating an efficiency of resource allocation by coordinating the objectives of the physician and the health care organization. Economically, the interests of the profession and the hospital must be synchronized. This model offers an approach to doing that very thing. It incorporates physician authority, respect, and societal dependence into the corporation, which is of value to the corporation and which certainly remains an objective of the profession. It resolves the conflict of management and the profession. It focuses the marketing efforts of the institution on the health care consumer rather than on the health care provider, as is so often the case now with hospitals as they attempt to make themselves attractive to physicians who are the gatekeepers to the hospital. It resolves the "turf" battle of physicians and hospitals. It clearly defines competitors in the medical marketplace, competitors who are health care corporations built upon a strong relationship and a durable commitment of the medical profession to the corporation.

Is there anything feasible to this response on the part of the medical profession? There are some things that would lead us to believe it is so. There are working models, such as the Cleveland

Clinic Foundation and Hospital, the Oschner Clinic, Straub Hospital and Clinic, Scripps Clinic and Research Hospital, and my own Lovelace Medical Foundation. I have had the opportunity to look at most of these institutions in recent years, and I am impressed by several things. They are big and they are getting bigger. They are successful and they are highly optimistic about the future. This is in contrast to other segments of the medical profession, certainly in our community, where declining income is characteristic; loss of market share is a reality; concern over the future is epidemic; and the love-hate relationship of the great partnership grows more intense every day.

I believe it is feasible because physicians, hospital management, and boards are very worried. Throughout this country we hear of hospital administrators and board members wringing their hands, proclaiming that the medical profession and the hospital must work together or both will suffer together. In my view this is absolutely true. The questions are, how do we do it? and is it feasible?

It is feasible because the profession has been committed to maintenance of quality in the health care organizations they serve, and it will continue to be. It is feasible because physicians are capable of learning about organizational affairs and mastering the art and science of management. I think that physicians will do well in positions of management and control of health care organizations because they are entrepreneurial. Physicians are very competitive and that will be essential to the success of health care corporations.

It is equally true that there are many obstacles to the physician-centered health care corporation. A major one is the paucity of physician organizations. Most of those in existence are group practice models that remain the minority type of medical practice. To meet the demand, great growth will be required. In addition, other types of physician-managed organizations must evolve.

This concept certainly flies in the face of fundamental values, beliefs, and economic commitments of the medical profession. There is an unquestionable and long-standing distrust of the health care organization by physicians. The evidence of past successes on the part of the medical profession in controlling health care organizations is very persuasive that it will continue in the future. The political and economic power of the medical profession remains highly potent. It is safe to say that a significant fraction of the medical profession still feels it can work its will on the health care organization and maintain the status quo. This is a distinct obstacle to change.

An initiative such as I have proposed is a threat to the hospital administration profession. Physicians unquestionably lack the skills and training that will be necessary if they are to assume more management responsibility in the health care organization. Once their skills are developed, however, with their knowledge of the health care process, they will become very capable administrators. They will predictably have a degree of credibility with physicians rarely enjoyed by nonphysician executives.

Finally, I think it is fair to say that there is a major reservoir of distrust of the medical profession by other health care professionals, such as nurses, and by hospital trustees, who probably would fear that the doctors may run any organization in which they have influence to serve the interest of the medical profession.

In conclusion, there is intense demand for change in the health care business today. I suggested to you that the status quo has failed and that the corporate or organizational solution is a likely response to the failure of the status quo. I have concluded that the present situation is one of gross, possibly irreconcilable conflict between the values and objectives of the medical profession and the agenda of both society and the hospital. It is these factors that have brought us to "the crossroads." It is my conclusion that a new health care organization centered on and managed by the medical profession is a likely path to a solution.

Henry Ford Hospital:
A Hospital-Sponsored Medical Group

STANLEY R. NELSON

I interpret my charge to be that of presenting essentially what amounts to a case study of the organization I represent because it has some relevancy to the subject that we're talking about today. It's hard to find similar models in the field. I think there are some that come close, but nothing precisely like this particular model. I think it would be very difficult to replicate the Henry Ford Hospital complex today.

A brief historical review of Henry Ford Hospital might prove helpful in understanding its present organizational structure. In a very real sense, the corporate name is misleading because, while the organization does maintain and operate a 1,000-bed hospital, a major portion of its efforts and resources are devoted to the management and operation of a very large, multispecialty group practice.

The hospital was established during World War I. A citizens' group was engaged in the process of developing a hospital for Detroit and the southeast Michigan community, and had solicited the participation of Henry Ford as treasurer of the development committee. If you are familiar with Henry Ford's philosophy and style, you know that he did not have a high regard for the efficiency of committees, so when the project encountered difficulties, he offered to repay all donations to that point and build a hospital for the community. The only condition he attached was that he run it. His offer was accepted.

This presented him with the challenge of managing a new kind of enterprise and, not surprisingly, he brought his distinctive organizational talents to bear on the opportunity. He had already made major contributions to American industrial techniques through the development and refinement of mass production processes and, of more significance for the hospital, had developed a passion for self-sufficiency and a high degree of integration in his industrial empire.

It is natural that these instincts and this philosophy should carry over to his hospital. Therefore, as he set about the process of opening this hospital, it was logical that the physicians should be an integral part. To his way of thinking this would be a more efficient way of providing hospital and medical services. The physicians could concentrate on what they do best: take care of patients. The hospital would provide the resources and support systems to enhance the physician. The proximity of physicians to beds, laboratories, and diagnostic technology would increase their effectiveness.

Unencumbered by any concerns for the prevailing attitudes toward group practice or salaried medical staffs, he went to Johns Hopkins and engaged a core of leading physicians and organized them into a hospital-based group practice.

To him, this made eminent sense. It was an efficient way of delivering health services; of integrating the physicans in the hospital; and of removing all the encumbrances of medical practice and management practice from the physicians and putting them in close proximity to the beds, to the laboratories, and to the diagnostic technology that they needed. He would, in turn, provide all of the support systems and resources that they needed to do their job.

Since this was a community hospital in every sense of the word, and since this was prior to the development of health insurance and third-party funding, he subsidized the hospital enterprise during the twenties and thirties. Since the Ford Motor Company did not become a public corporation until 1956, he could support the hospital directly from the company. The archives of the Ford Company contain a ledger sheet titled "Mr. Ford's Hospital," which identifies the annual subsidy required to balance the books.

Given this background, Henry Ford Hospital today has the appearance of and, indeed, functions very much like, other large multispecialty group practices. While virtually every other similar organization has its origins in a successful group practice that ultimately developed a hospital to meet its requirements, the reverse is true in our case.

Bringing this organizational pattern into the present time presents an interesting range of advantages and some disadvantages. There are several advantages. First, this type of organization presents a great opportunity for the efficient use of professional resources; that is, the opportunity to balance specialty and subspecialty resources against need. In addition, as we have developed multiple delivery sites, it is possible to deploy specialized professional manpower in fractional units; if an orthopedist is needed two days a week at a given site, this can usually be provided.

Second, the close relationship of physicians to hospital makes it easier to deal with alternative delivery systems and respond expeditiously to a changing environment. We have been able to do this in the area of comprehensive, offsite ambulatory care, HMOs, and capitated prepayment programs.

Third, cost containment measures are potentially easier to achieve when the hospital and physician are tightly integrated. We feel we have been able to address DRG decisions more effectively because of our structure.

Fourth, it may be easier for our type of organization to shape itself for changing market circumstances or opportunities. This is true in the area of emphasizing certain subspecialties.

Fifth, this type of organization avoids duplications in capital asset allocation, i.e., the physician group is not duplicating hardware or technology provided by the hospital as sometimes occurs in other settings.

Sixth, the interrelationships between clinical practice, education, and research can be quite readily adjusted in this type of structure.

Seventh, decisions typically can be made expeditiously, at least in comparison with university hospital settings.

Eighth, the inherent group loyalty encompasses the hospital and provides a stability that eliminates some concerns present elsewhere.

There are some disadvantages inherent in this organizational pattern also. First, dynamic tensions exist with respect to how decisions are made, how resources are allocated, how new programs are identified, and how key professional staff are identified. These tend to be time-consuming. A corollary is that governance arrangements require constant tuning.

Second, hospitals have a different set of regulatory requirements from individual physicians, and our type of organization carries that added burden.

Third, a group of employed physicians (in a world of independent physicians) presents certain limits in the ability to relate to other organizations.

Fourth, group loyalties and institutional responsibilities sometimes make it difficult to change directions by eliminating programs. It is painful to remove a "member of the family."

Fifth, some physicians are not comfortable with the concept of growth which is important to a viable enterprise, and they may tend to slow us down some.

Sixth, perceptions of equitable compensation are difficult to achieve. The process, inevitably, involves subjective judgments about contributions to the organization. It is my perception that the perfect compensation plan has not yet been devised for a physician group or for any professional group.

Perhaps the attitude of the typical physician we attract reflects the nature of our organization and some of the reasons why a physician would commit his professional career to Henry Ford Hospital. High on the list is a prevailing attitude that our multispecialty group offers an excellent way to practice quality medicine. The ongoing and easy access to other specialties within the group and the peer review inherent in a common medical record are appealing. The readily available support systems, which remove many of the problems of private practice, and the opportunity for a more predictable and structured life-style are also added attractions.

The opportunity for meaningful teaching as an integral part of a physician's professional life is a high priority item. These opportunities are available through seventeen residency programs and a complement of 402 house officers as well as extensive undergraduate teaching at the third- and fourth-year levels with University of Michigan Medical School students, some of whom spend their entire third and fourth years at Henry Ford Hospital.

The opportunity to participate in or relate to ongoing clinical research programs that are relevant to physicians' professional interests is a very attractive feature. There are thirty-one different research programs staffed by 155 research personnel. They are professionally stimulating and provide an added dimension to a physician's professional life.

In conclusion, the typical physician in this group will say that if he were not at Henry Ford Hospital, he would probably be in a university medical center. From this it is quite apparent that our kind of organization attracts a physician who is somewhat different from the norm, one who has special interests and needs and affords this kind of organization with an interesting array of advantages, disadvantages, opportunities, and challenges.

Henry Ford Hospital is reasonably well designed for the current market. In spite of some very difficult environmental problems, we have been and continue to be able to respond to what major purchasers of health care are seeking.

Doctors Create a Corporation to Deal with a Hospital

JOSEPH F. BOYLE, M.D.

As a result of the burgeoning economic, legislative, and legal pressures now bearing down on hospitals and the resulting interhos-
pital conflicts, a number of hospital medical staffs have incorporated or are planning to incorporate to strengthen their position
in dealing with hospital governing boards. The theory is that
when conflicts arise, the medical staff would thus become one
corporate entity dealing with another, the hospital.

The hospital staff where I practice does have a separate corporation, and that corporation has separate officers and separate articles of incorporation and bylaws than the hospital medical staff
organization, which continues to provide governance for the staff
within the hospital under the jurisdiction of the hospital board of
trustees, who are responsible for the operation of that hospital.

Quite recently it was proposed that the hospital and the medical staff become involved in contracting with an organization of
PPOS in southern California. They proposed to put together
twenty-one prestigious hospitals and staffs in a single entity that
would offer services transportable over a three-county area. The
first requirement was that the hospital staff had to have an entity
that could contract for that staff. Most hospitals were faced with
the question of putting together a corporate entity, a limited partnership, a full partnership, or some other legal body that could
participate in these negotiations which ultimately led to the formation of this twenty-one hospital and hospital medical staff
group.

The hospital where I practice has had a corporation for twenty-
one years, with its own officers, and was capable of saying, "Yes,
the president is now authorized to go and participate in these discussions and become a member of the board of directors of the

multiple PPO organization." This is just one example of what can be done.

However, there is no magic in incorporation. A corporation is treated like an artificial person under the law, but so is a partnership, a voluntary unincorporated association, or a joint venture. As for medical staff activities to advance its own self interest—but not in conflict with objectives of good patient care—it is immaterial whether it is incorporated or unincorporated. In both instances, the medical staff will be treated as an entity, particularly in dealings with the hospital governing board.

Incorporation indicates that the organized medical staff wants to be recognized as a separate entity. Whether it calls itself a voluntary membership association or not, it can act as a corporate entity. So incorporation adds nothing in terms of so acting.

There can be disadvantages to the medical staff if it incorporates. The very fact that it is separately incorporated could increase its exposure to professional liability suits, because it would be the corporation that would be responsible for making certain each member of the medical staff met the standards established for quality patient care.

For example, a medical staff corporation could be held liable for the negligence of an individual staff member if it knew or should have known that the member was not competent to perform certain patient care procedures and the patient then suffers an injury for which damages are sought. Such suits usually name the hospital but, by holding itself a separate entity, the medical staff corporation also could be named. And if damages are awarded, the hospital might then seek indemnification from the medical staff corporation.

The AMA believes hospital medical staffs do have a right to protect their interests, so we are encouraging them to arrange for their own legal counsels. But here, too, there are pitfalls. Such attorneys should not be hired purely in an adversarial sense, which could raise antitrust questions. Such attorneys should consider the interests of both the medical staff and the hospital. For that reason, we recommend that any attorney hired by a medical staff should have medical as well as legal experience. An attorney already retained by a county or metropolitan medical society or attorneys who also have an M.D. degree are two alternatives.

Examining the reasons behind the tidal wave of litigation surrounding hospital medical staffs can be both educational and beneficial.

The courts have not attempted to determine which physicians should have staff privileges at which hospital. But the large number of suits filed during the past twenty years or so has educated judges on issues related to staff privileges and how "due process" operates in hospitals. What has brought about this increase in litigation? There are two primary legal doctrines involved.

The first holds that hospitals must assure patients of a safe environment and quality care during their hospital stay.

The second doctrine recognizes that a hospital cannot remain open unless it can assure patients of skilled and specialized medical services. But it cannot arbitrarily decide which physicians should have medical staff privileges that are indispensable to modern medical practice.

So the hospital faces a quandary in making sure it doesn't incur liability for the negligent selection or retention of staff physicians, while simultaneously assuring physicians of the substantive and procedural safeguards under fundamental fairness or "due process."

But the hospital has had lots of help in addressing the quandary. Physicians have been busy writing into medical staff bylaws due process hearing provisions and procedures to carry out the provisions. Hospital attorneys have been even busier making legally certain that a staff physician will be afforded so much due process that a court can find nothing to overturn once the hospital proceedings have ended.

The motto is, "give the physician so much due process that no court will interfere." The way this is done can be mind-boggling. In 1971 the Joint Commission on Accreditation of Hospitals revised its hospital accreditation standards, moving from minimum to optimal achievable standards. JCAH then assembled a committee of attorneys familiar with hospital law to modify fair hearing procedures for physicians whose staff privileges have been curtailed, suspended, or revoked. A JCAH staff member then diagrammed the procedural steps. The diagram looked like it had been drawn by Rube Goldberg.

The tragedy is that these due process procedures can result in as much as eighteen months of hearings at the hospital level alone. And all too often very little may be accomplished, except perhaps the fomenting of a great deal of bitterness between the accused and the accusers.

Let's consider an extreme example. A physician with privileges in obstetrics and gynecology is charged with using abusive language with nurses, not using proper sterile techniques, and failing to comply with hospital policies on the presence of prospective fathers in the labor and delivery rooms. The hearing begins following suspension of his staff privileges. The physician retains legal counsel for the hearing at the medical staff level and the hospital calls in its attorney.

Nurses testify that the physician used abusive language, and charge that the physician failed to use sterile rubber gloves during a procedure three years earlier.

The physician then brings in witnesses who testify that an emergency bleeding problem developed and the physician shouted at the nurse for not providing the necessary equipment and supplies he had ordered.

The panel of medical staff members listens to the testimony and the physician's response to the other charges filed against him. The panel then goes into executive session and recommends that additional charges be added. The first hearing lasts twelve hours over a period of four evenings.

When the physician receives written notice of the second set of charges, certified mail, return receipt requested, a second hearing is held. This continues at evening sessions for another three months. When the findings are adverse, the hearing moves to the appellate stage before the full hospital governing board.

By this time, the physician has been excluded from the hospital for nine months, and has built a birthing center in his home. Now the physician is ready to sue the hospital, and the hospital is ready to try the license revocation process. Trial begins and the physician brings in an expert witness from a prestigious university hospital department of obstetrics and gynecology. The witness convinces the court that the physician's techniques and treatments met the standards of the university hospital.

So the court orders the hospital to permit the physician to reapply for staff privileges. Back at the hospital, positions have solidified into dead-set opposition to the regranting of privileges. When the application is denied, the entire hearing process is repeated at the hospital level.

The physician has now been without privileges for three years, and is distraught because his professional reputation has been blemished. He's convinced there's a conspiracy to run him out of town.

What does he do? He hires another attorney and files another suit against the hospital. This time he goes to federal court rather than the state court and alleges a violation of antitrust laws. This is a tempting option for both physician and attorney, because a victorious claimant not only has staff privileges restored but recovers three times the amount of damages claimed.

As might be expected, however, the court rules no antitrust violation occurred since restraining the trade of one physician does not significantly affect interstate commerce. The courts are generally convinced that antitrust laws were not written to assure that individual physicians have an adequate number of patients or to specify in what settings such physicians should provide treatment.

The process has now dragged on for nine years. The physician is now acting as his own attorney, and decides new legal avenues should be explored to set the record straight. So he files another suit in state court, charging that the hospital attorney had a conflict of interest in representing the hospital and that the judge in the first court hearing should have been disqualified since he is related to the hospital attorney.

When the physician loses, he appeals and succeeds in getting an order for a new trial from the appellate court on the grounds that the first judge should have excused himself.

Back again to the hospital where attitudes have grown even more adamant. It offers the physician $100,000 to drop legal proceedings and set up practice in Australia. The physician turns around and files suit against the hospital attorney, charging misuse of hospital funds.

This story has no end. There is still a pending action in the case that began nine years ago, and now the physician is challenging the bench of the state supreme court.

But the lesson for hospital medical staffs should be clear. Objective, honest peer review of the clinical performance of physicians should minimize the need for a physician whose privileges are revoked for incompetence to seek redress in the courts. If a medical staff recommends revocation to reduce competition, or because of personal dislikes, due process at the hospital level won't have the magic that hospital attorneys rely upon.

Related judicial trends have other lessons to teach. Hospital and medical staff bylaws place the responsibility for credentialing and review directly on the medical staff. Then the law says the hospital governing board is responsible if proper standards of care are not met. So courts are finding that the ultimate responsibility for quality assurance rests with governing boards, and that the hospital and its medical staff are an inseparable entity that serves the community, as well as patients. The courts also have been willing to support hospital peer review and quality assurance programs under due process.

This has created a new group of legal specialists in preventive hospital law. They teach hospital governing boards to put into writing all of the possible legalese associated with actions against physicians, including the entire hearing and appeals process.

This can transform a hearing into a legal swamp for physicians, because rulings on what can be accepted as evidence, how much proof is needed, and who has the burden of proof are the province of lawyers, not physicians. In one case cited as a model of due process, the hearing panel was chaired by an experienced attorney. The physician involved was presented with written charges supported by ninety-five hospital documents. A hearing transcript by a court reporter was made, and an opportunity for an appeal to the full hospital governing board was afforded. So the long legal process began.

Fortunately, more hospital staff physicians and trustees are coming to realize the process seems to be unduly complicated, time consuming, traumatic, and expensive, and has more to do with good law than good medicine. It also tends to institutionalize and cement the attitudes of the hospitals and physicians involved, when a less rigid proceeding, at least for the first hearing, might produce better results and fairer treatment.

Less legalism would promote more justice in terms of determining real clinical competence, and not tend to stifle it or bury it under a mountain of procedural niceties.

The very legal problems that tend to splinter intrahospital relationships also may very well end up cementing those relationships. And that is of the utmost importance. The legal view of a hospital and its medical staff as a single, inseparable entity could well do much more good than harm. Because the truth is, one cannot exist without the other, not in this modern world of medicine. For legal reasons, hospitals and medical staffs are working harder together to assure quality care, and in risk management to prevent needless patient injury.

This need to act together, to regard the hospital and medical staff as a single entity, is being strongly reinforced by those social, economic, and legislative forces which I cited at the outset.

We are being asked to make hospital care more cost-effective, while maintaining its quality and availability, and to do so within the economic constraints of the new prospective pricing, or diagnosis related group, reimbursement system under Medicare. And this kind of system could be imposed on all medical services, including those provided in physicians' offices, if some people in the Congress have their way.

This makes it all the more imperative that hospital staff physicians, administrators, and trustees work much harder together if we are to survive together. That's the only way we *can* survive together. And survive we must, for the sake of patients first of all.

Doctors and Hospital Form a Cooperative Organization

PAUL M. ELLWOOD, JR., M.D.

For the past year, InterStudy has been working with a select group of hospitals and their medical staffs, exploring and implementing one form of health care innovation—the medical staff-hospital joint venture, which we call "MeSH."

The idea has stirred much interest. Hundreds of organizations have contacted us to find out what MeSH is all about. Many hospitals and medical staffs have invited us to spend a few days exploring the concept with administrators, physicians, trustees, and business leaders in their communities. Yet only one group has progressed to the point of actually implementing one of these medical staff-hospital joint ventures.

We've been forced to recognize that the idea of hospitals and doctors getting together in a constructive, organized way—which to us appears very appealing and very logical—does not exert an irresistible force upon everyone. At times it seems as though we've run up against an immovable object. In part, the immovable object is a set of old assumptions about the way health-care organizations work. Hospitals and medical staffs are used to the idea of functioning separately. They accept as given a relationship that is symbiotic at best and antagonistic at worst. For physicians especially, professional identity is based on autonomy. They see the tradition of functioning alone tightly tied to their mission of controlling the quality of medical care.

Andrew Pettigrew, who has studied stragetic planning in organizations, observed that unsuccessful companies tend to cling to flagrantly faulty assumptions about the world for years after things begin to change; they pay little or no attention to signs of change around them or signals that they too should change. They ignore the fact that sometimes it's necessary to confront change, and sometimes it's tremendously advantageous to do so.

Still, it's difficult for a system bound by successful professional experience and tradition to change. It helps to be nudged. Often the most subtle and effective nudges come in the form of new language and new imagery that gives us a different perspective, an enlightening insight, or a fresh vision of the future. That's part of what I see as InterStudy's mission. We try to seed the health care system with new ideas, new language, and new imagery for the way things can work, like health maintenance organizations and preferred provider organizations. That's what this MeSH idea is all about. Throughout this paper, I'll use the word "MeSH" a lot. By using it, I don't mean to refer to any one rigid model but rather to the broader idea of a medical staff-hospital joint venture.

We've come to view MeSH as a measure of health care organizations' ability to remain flexible and respond innovatively in a rapidly changing environment. Our expectation is that those organizations that move now, either through MeSH or through a similar hospital-physician collaborative arrangement, to heal the traditional tensions and to position themselves for continuing change will be those most likely to win in the new medical-economic environment.

Rationale for MeSH

We designed MeSH based on the following four assumptions about the direction of health care.

First, fee-for-service, solo, and small group practice physicians and conventional hospitals are highly vulnerable in the new medical-economic environment, especially as the pace of change accelerates.

Second, as price competition intensifies, those organizations that survive will be comprehensive, vertically integrated health care organizations. They will resemble successful group practices in their ability to be selective about both the number and the abilities of participating physicians.

Third, payment methods will continue to change rapidly and unpredictably; all will put physicians and hospitals at risk for each other's behavior.

Fourth, as the needs of consumers shift and the number of physicians increases, conveniently located, around-the-clock satellite clinics will become increasingly important.

Confronted by these patterns of change, InterStudy sought an organizational model that would be both effective and acceptable.

We therefore designed MeSH to provide a framework for constructively addressing the financial and professional issues inherent in the changing environment, without gratuitously disrupting the status quo. In other words, MeSH is a measured, moderate response to change. Participating physicians and hospitals control the nature and extent of change to which they are exposed. Physicians can continue to practice out of their own offices on a fee-for-service basis; hospitals do not have to convert all of their revenues to prepaid or prospective payment. Neither the hospital nor the physician has to participate in any program not viewed as beneficial.

Flexibility is perhaps the MeSH model's greatest asset. We purposely designed MeSH to be as flexible as possible to enhance its applicability and acceptability. We considered flexibility critical to quick installment of the MeSH model, and we assumed speed of installation crucial in a rapidly changing environment.

The MeSH Model

In the MeSH model, a hospital and its medical staff create a new corporation. This discrete business entity (the MeSH) is *equally* owned by the hospital and those members of the medical staff who choose to participate. Thus, rights, responsibilities, and control are evenly balanced. Hospital and medical staff have equal voting power in stockholder and partnership meetings. They have equal representation on the governing board of the MeSH corporation. Equal initial investments are usually required from the physicians and the hospital.

MeSH is a multipurpose organization. The central MeSH corporation is responsible for many of the critical tasks in which the economic interests of doctors and hospitals overlap: coordination, financial risk avoidance, and utilization management systems. The MeSH model also provides for the creation of a series of subcorporations, or MeSHplans. Each MeSHplan can be designed around one of the following current health care opportunities (new MeSHplans can be designed as new opportunities present themselves): (1) prospective payment management (e.g., Medicare DRG); (2) price competitive medical plans (e.g., HMOS, PPOS); and (3) out-of-hospital health service ventures (e.g., ambulatory care satellite clinics, surgicenters, birthing centers, and home health care).

Each physician member of the central MeSH can choose which

MeSHplan(s) he or she wants to participate in. For example, if the MeSH sponsors a PPO each MeSH physician may choose either to provide services through the PPO or to stay out of that particular program.

InterStudy's Experience with MeSH

In the past year, InterStudy has spent two or more days exploring the MeSH concept in each of thirty hospitals. The hospitals and medical staffs interested in MeSH are a varied lot. We have worked with individual community hospitals and hospitals tied into multihospital systems. While we have worked with no investor-owned hospitals, we have discussed MeSH with hospitals associated with academic medical centers and multispecialty group practices. We have worked with hospitals in small towns as well as in large cities. Some have been in very liberal medical communities and some have been in conservative communities. Some have been in regulated states and some in highly competitive environments.

Of the thirty hospitals we have worked with, sixteen have moved beyond the initial educational and evaluative stage to work seriously on MeSH installation. While no MeSH is yet operational, the hospital and medical staff we have worked with the longest are rapidly approaching that point. Franklin County Public Hospital in Greenfield, Massachusetts, has begun enrolling doctors in what they hope will become the nation's first operational MeSH.

Barriers to MeSH

We've been working with the MeSH idea for more than a year. Why, after all this time, is Franklin Hospital the only group close to implementing a medical staff-hospital joint venture? What's the problem? What has taken so long? In the course of considering the MeSH idea in hospitals and medical staffs across the country, we've begun to notice some patterns. Based on our experience, we can now identify several major barriers to implementing a hospital-physician joint venture. All of these barriers stem from the traditional pattern of interaction between hospitals and physicians to which I referred earlier. Hospitals and physicians have rarely had to work together on the business aspects of the practice of medicine. They are not used to doing it. They are not used to thinking about it. It is therefore extremely difficult to get them together.

In some hospitals we've worked in, a strong-willed, controlling administrator has been the barrier. Such administrators refuse to give any semblance of control to physicians, whom they regard as divided and unreliable. In other instances, it has been the hospitals or the medical society that blocked the joint venture idea. They distrust the hospital and oppose becoming any closer to it out of fear of becoming controlled by it. Some hospitals and medical staffs have sought "safer," less innovative responses to change. For example, attracted by the idea of strength in numbers, one hospital decided that joining a horizontally integrated multihospital system was the most effective and least risky way to relieve economic pressures.

Traditionally, hospitals have been more apt to strike treaties with other hospitals than to compete aggressively. Some hospitals and doctors have viewed the price-competitive plans that MeSH may establish as a declaration of war on their fellow hospitals and doctors even in communities where outside health-care firms are entering their markets. The advantage that outsiders enjoy is that they have no established relationships within the health community to protect; as a result, the majority of the new competitive plans end up being controlled by others than the existing health-care organizations.

Some hospitals and medical staffs have looked at the hospital-physician joint venture idea as unwarranted overreaction. Their feeling was that despite some changes, there were as yet no serious threats to the status quo. They feared that they would only accelerate change by taking action to anticipate it and preferred instead to passively resist change for as long as possible. In many cases, we encountered a lack of effective leadership in both the hospital administration and medical staff. The lack of physician leadership was a particularly difficult barrier, since doctors are more numerous and more divided and lack any mechanism for reaching consensus. Compounding the barriers just mentioned has been a general atmosphere of uncertainty. Providers have been unwilling to get involved in a venture around which there are so many unresolved technical questions. Associations representing providers haven't known what advice to give their constituencies. Health-care consultants have been caught off guard and are unprepared to address a restructured health-care system.

We've encountered several practical barriers in the course of actually installing MeSH organizations. First, legal uncertainties: there is a lack of relevant case law and the new organizational arrangements raise difficult questions related to antitrust issues, corporate practice, and classification of the new health plans as insurers or providers. Second, lack of management personnel who are both qualified and perceived as being unbiased: HMOs have snapped up available medical managers knowledgeable about incentive systems and drawing management from either the hospital or the medical staff is seen as tilting the MeSH in favor of that side. Third, unavailability of management information systems that can simultaneously cope with a full range of reimbursement systems plus the qualitative dimension of patient care. Although this is a problem throughout the health care system, it has surfaced repeatedly in MeSH negotiations. Fourth, lack of insurers or brokers who can provide access to employee markets for combined hospitals and medical staffs.

Incentives for MeSH

In those organizations that have avoided or overcome the barriers described above, we have identified two key factors for progressing with the joint venture idea.

In every instance, those who have gone ahead with MeSH have done so, at least in part, because of their perception of the impending threat of competitive forces: other hospitals and physicians as well as HMO, PPO, surgicenters, and other ventures. The driving force for these doctors and hospitals has been a very serious concern about gaining and retaining patients and filling hospital beds. This concern far outweighs any interest in collaborating to hit the DRG prospective payment rates.

In every instance where MeSH is moving, effective leadership has been as vital an ingredient as competition. On the surface, setting up a joint venture appears to be a defensive move by shrewd hospitals and physicians in highly competitive environments. While this impression is valid, it is not complete. My belief is that the health-care leaders who have most actively promoted MeSH have also had an unstated, hidden agenda. While few have articulated these ideas, my opinion is that they believe there is something positive to be gained from restructuring the traditional hospital-medical staff relationship. They believe that a joint venture will enable them to provide better quality care. They believe that the joint venture approach will lead to more cost-effective and accessible care, delivered by a very select and cohesive group of providers. While the mob may want only to hold their own competitively, the real leaders are motivated by a desire to express a set of firmly held values.

Conclusion

After more than a year of working with MeSH, I am very optimistic about the idea. It will be applied in various forms in many if not most of the country's hospitals. In fact, based on the relatively minor role that I've seen existing hospitals and doctors play in shaping their futures, I believe MeSH is more important than ever. It's a logical step for hospitals and physicians to take; but it's a difficult one because of the absence of precedent.

To make the MeSH idea work, to be able to take that difficult step, strong leadership is needed. This has been our experience with the hospitals and physicians that have chosen to go ahead with MeSH. In every case, they have been led by creative and pragmatic individuals who see in change not threats but rather opportunities for themselves, for their organizations, and for an improved health-care system. On a superficial level, they are experts at motivating others by paying lip service to the necessity of responding to changes imposed by external forces; on a deeper level, they are compelled by a conviction that the new ways of organizing medical care are not just necessary but can actually be better. Perhaps they are simply less hampered than others by the mechanical pictures of the way things work that most people carry around in their heads.

Still, there are limits to what these leaders can accomplish by themselves. To forge an integrated health-care system, I'm convinced that leaders from all segments of the industry must work together. I'm encouraged by opportunities like Duke University's Private Sector Conference, which each year gives health care leaders a forum for talking and listening to one another. Perhaps if we do a good job of communicating, we can jostle some of our old assumptions about one another and together shape a new culture.

For my part, I would like to leave you with an image of the future borrowed from the medical leaders we have worked with on MeSH. In the face of change, they are not clinging desperately to old behaviors or harping about new constraints or burrowing in defensively. They are moving ahead positively, convinced that the way things have been in the past is not necessarily the best of all possible worlds. They perceive a better future and will shape one. Their leadership is sure and excellent, a precedent for all of us.

Discussion

MR. NELSON: I want to attack Dave Ottensmeyer on his monopoly of management in the province of physicians. I would submit that there's nothing sacred or magic about physician-managers any more than there is on the other side of the corner. I think that's been demonstrated amply in other types of organizations and in other industries. The whole Harvard Business School is predicated on the principle that management techniques are transferable to different settings.

DR. OTTENSMEYER: The point about physician-chief executive officers was only to establish an extreme. The thing that's wrong with the health care of the typical hospital is that the medical profession has refused to be involved in the management of the health-care organization and hospital administrators have likewise worked to be sure that they're not involved. There's nothing magic about putting physicians in those places, but I think it's a mistake not to have physicians involved in the process. I think it's a timely maneuver right now to move very forcibly in that direction, which we have avoided doing in the past.

DR. BOYLE: If one is intent at the beginning to develop some totally new and restructured system, the probabilities are that we're unlikely to respond to needs in a more informed fashion than in the past. As you go about trying to create cooperative endeavors to resolve very real problems and respond to the cries of help from people around us, it's best that you not ask people to do something that you're not going to do in the first place.

DR. B. L. RHODES: When it comes to the great partnership, the Kaiser Health Plan stands on both sides, or perhaps more accurately, in the middle. In our first five regions we own and operate our own hospitals. We contract with those hospitals and with independent medical groups to provide care for our members. We tied the hospitals' and medical groups' financial success together, as we felt this might be an additional incentive toward the creation of mutually beneficial and cooperative relationships between the two and, indeed, we believe it has. With this arrangement, we have been able to control the utilization of all of our resources in a reasonably satisfactory fashion.

In the next four regions that we established, we deal with community hospitals. We hospitalize our members in community hospitals, and our medical groups have to deal with these community hospitals. I'm pleased to say that we've also been able to perform to our mutual benefit in that situation. We've been able to control the utilization of our resources approximately as well as we have in our own hospitals. We have had an occasional administrator in a community hospital say to us that he can see some increase in acuity in our patients and perhaps instead of paying less we should be paying more than the average community rate, or the daily rate. Be that as it may, we feel that the relationships have been good.

We do feel that organized groups of physicians who are fully responsible for all aspects of the care of their patients are in a somewhat better position to negotiate and maintain such arrangements with the community hospitals than are individual solo practitioners.

When it comes to DRGs, we aren't certain how threatened we are by them. In all probability, in the beginning at least, we will do rather well in our own hospitals with the DRG arrangements, that is at least until such time as DRG payments are reduced, which we fully believe they will be.

We've had no problems yet with the community hospitals over the DRG arrangement, but we can anticipate the possibility of a closed staff and we certainly don't plan to move any services out of those hospitals in order to maintain our relationships with them.

When we had only one hospital, the physicians owned and operated the hospital. That is no longer the case. Our doctors have created corporations and partnerships to deal with community hospitals and with the Kaiser Health Plan. We certainly haven't found a perfect system. We're still looking.

DR. ELLWOOD: That comment raises a critical question that our panel raised too, and that is whether the issue here is organizing physicians to practice together or forming a close relationship between doctors and hospitals. Each of the joint ventures or each of the corporations described is where physicians own hospitals or where hospitals own physicians. The key characteristic is that that's group practice which carefully uses a set of doctors. So, what is the critical ingredient here?

DR. BOYLE: The corporation that we have at the Good Samaritan Hospital was formed with the assistance and support and encouragement of hospital's top management which is critical to operate a close relationship at any place that I know of. That is the objective.

DR. WILBUR: In these presentations, the first two speakers spoke to doctors who belong to the group and doctors who don't, carefully selected in both cases. The last two speakers appeared to take in all the members of a current hospital staff. The observation I have is that in these models that you presented you have no system for removing outlier physicians, the ones who are not cost effective.

Dr. Sammons said earlier that we're going to see closed hospital staffs. Are they going to be closed on the basis of quality, on the basis of who's there now? Are they going to be closed on the basis of who is the cheapest or who's the most cost effective physician? If so, what happens to good physicians who, for one reason or another, are frozen out from hospital privileges in a given community because they're considered cost-ineffective, or maybe just not the kind of people we want to associate with in that closed hospital staff?

DR. BOYLE: That is one of the benefits we're going to have in organizing an established entity to deal with those questions. If you are now being asked by a broker for PPOs or some other such entity to enter into such negotiations with them, they're going to be concerned with utilization review. That group obviously should be concerned about quality of care. But in my own personal view that kind of review of physician practice should be a function of the organized medical staff. The corporation may or may not include all the members of that staff.

DR. ELLWOOD: We've seen a proliferation of changes of hospital bylaws such that hospitals are giving themselves the right to exclude and remove physicians from the staff who fail to practice cost-effective medicine. In the MeSH model it's impossible to be selective about physicians beyond membership in the medical staff. Legally it is very difficult to have sufficient grounds for being selective and technically it is very difficult to do so.

The usual set of doctors on the hospital medical staff has opinions about who practices conservative medicine, but in most instances they don't really know. They also don't know whether they can change physicians' behavior once they come into a new arrangement. I would tend to opt for their being open about these matters at the outset but recognize that with the passage of time everything is subject to the competitive environment. They will have the right to become increasingly selective and to remove certain physicians from the group who jeopardize the rest of the members of the group or the hospital by their styles of practice.

DR. OTTENSMEYER: If you had to set out and design and put into existence one of these competitive models in a crowded community like Albuquerque, where there are too many physicians and too many beds and they're out building more just to use funds, how would you do it if you had your choice?

I think the organization in which you can select the physicians and in which you can design the practice and the product and package it and price it the way you want it and communicate the way you desire has to be effective. A very clear story can be told by going up and looking at Henry Ford Hospital. It has gone through some tough times going back to the changes that occurred in the late sixties and the early seventies in which they were able to adapt an organization, completely restructured, and move in a different direction. Few institutions could have responded that well.

MR. NELSON: It seems to me that your trade-off here is between the organizational ideal and political reality, what's achievable. Depending on where you fall out on that scale, you'd better be far enough up the scale so that there can be some behavior change. I think that's why you see things like IPAS go down the sewer—because nothing changes. They create a structure and a financing mechanism and nothing else happens and so it fails.

DR. ROGERS: The theme that I hear running through the comments is basic physician distrust of organizations with entrepreneurial styles and distrust of hospitals. With a few exceptions, maybe we're in the wrong generation to talk about it. We've all been thirty years or so in the business while the young people who are now coming out are really quite a different creature. By 1990, 40 percent of the practicing physicians will have graduated post-1978. That's a great big change.

In talking with those young people, I find they are much less entrepreneurial. They are much more comfortable with salaried kinds of slots. They are much more used to working in groups than all of us were. Some of the kinds of changes that have been suggested here may come a lot faster than we think because there's a whole new set of creatures who don't quite sound like us who are now labeled "physicians."

DR. ELLWOOD: The dilemma is that you have to shape the health system around what is there right now: the power structure, the medical staff, and such.

DR. BOYLE: All the survey data we have indicate that things are going in precisely the opposite direction. The younger, more recent graduates are becoming more conservative, are less likely to accept a salary, are more likely to be interested in small group practices. That is a change in the trend that has been going on for five or six years.

In most hospitals and communities that I've seen today, the leaders are younger physicians. In fact, in most county medical societies today the leaders are young physicians. Santa Barbara County, one of the oldest, most established medical communities, has an association president who has been in practice for only four and a half years.

DR. NELSON: Can physicians live without the hospitals? And why would they want to try? First, the hospital is threatening the doctor with a corporate image he doesn't particularly like. Second, the hospital is more and more a place of a lot of hassle. It's not a pleasant place to work. A lot of paperwork and records and house staff and pushy nurses and inadequate parking. Third, increased professional liability. Fourth, inadequate compensation for the time spent.

I've roughly calculated for the hospital care that I've delivered in the last year, if you include transportation time, and it works out to $25 an hour. A lot of self-respecting farmers won't work for that.

If the question might be answered yes, I would like to live without the hospital, the corollary to that is, could I live without the hospital? In primary care it would be easy. I'd do about 98 percent of my work outside the hospital. I have a laboratory and x rays and I can deliver biopsies and endoscopy all outside the hospital and I'll gladly refer critical care problems to a full-time hospital physician because my ego doesn't need crises. The only problem is the time my patients want me most is when they're most ill. Consequently, I don't always have that choice.

Now, surgical care is another matter. A lot can be done in the surgicenter; all they have to do is put together a three-day convalescent unit attached to it and I suspect that a lot of work by surgeons could be done outside the hospital.

Well, what would the hospital then become? Imagine a 500-bed facility with 300 empty beds and 200 intensive care beds all full, an exclusive full-time staff who are underworked and underpaid because they're salaried and they work about the kind of hours that I worked when I was in the Air Force. The costs per occupied bed are astronomical and the relations between physicians and patients aren't very good because they didn't know each other before they got really sick. The per patient liability costs, of course, are huge.

Is all that farfetched? Not terribly so! For primary care specialties, it's entirely feasible, and I don't think a lot of change would have to take place in the way surgeons do business to really bring that scenario about.

PROFESSOR LIPSCOMB: I was listening with interest when Dr. Ellwood was talking in the earlier part of his comments about the economic and social reasons why MeSH would be succeeding. Then he got to the punch line which is that it's barely moving!

He listed a number of good institutional reasons to expect that, but he said places where it would work or flourish are those where there is intense competition and also some strong leadership. Leadership is quixotic but competition is not, and it may be coming with greater force in certain areas than we see.

The DRGs are here but that's only a small thing. There is talk of all-payer systems. There is talk of extending the DRG system so that the hospital and the physician are paid jointly. There is talk of tightening DRGs and having a slower rate of increase in its prices than people had first thought.

We also have an increasing supply of physician manpower still coming along. There are a lot of factors in the market whose full forces have not been felt yet which might make it a bit more hospitable for some of these arrangements to provide for a streamlined competing organization.

DR. ELLWOOD: This problem of the quixotic nature of leadership is crucial. This is the reason why the national health care firms are sweeping across the country. One year ago, Orlando didn't have a single national medical care corporation. It now has five of them and every one of them is a branch of a national firm. None of them was started by people connected with the health system in Orlando.

During its early days, the whole HMO movement had social, entrepreneurial people who started these things randomly distributed across the country. Now, we have these national organizations, with strong leadership and strong financing, which pick out the best places to go and go there regardless of what's there already.

MR. SHELTON: What I hear described sounds like a technique for hospitals and, to a lesser degree, for physicians to protect their market share. I would be interested in more comments on how these arrangements would deal with unnecessary utilization and reduction of excess capacity in the community. If each facility in the community adopted a program such as has been described, I can see costs going through the ceiling by the end of the year.

MR. MCNERNEY: Dr. Ellwood said at one point that the lack of access to market was one of the inhibiting factors in the development of the MeSH program. After you put the doctors and the hospitals together in a cohesive, vibrant, exciting whole, how do you go to market? Does that whole make sense? Is it salable to employers and to others, or does it introduce the need of joining with other institutions in order to combine quality and reasonable access?

DR. DUVAL: It occurred to me that while our past was characterized by having the patient pay a fee to a physician to make all the decisions, the future is going to be characterized by the government determining what level of care will be distributed and where and what facilities there will be, by PROs deciding what standards will be applied, by business determining which problems will be covered, by payers deciding what a diagnosis is worth, and by alternative delivery systems saying where the patient will get the services and what kind of services.

I guess my concern is whether we are being pushed to a preoccupation with structure or process or organization or financing such that we may overlook the patient we're serving.

DR. BOYLE: That's what I think it's all about. As long as we make certain that the directions we are attempting to shape in the future for delivering medical care and hospital care and the health services provide people with the widest opportunities for access to excellence, then we are going to prevail. If our concerns are more personal and selfish, then we're going to fail.

DR. OTTENSMEYER: If you go back and look at the socioeconomic writings of the twenties and thirties, everybody said that group medical practice was rational and the logical thing to do. It obviously would be the key to organizing health care delivery services in this country. One of the things we may see now is an acceleration of the formation of groups simply because there will be somebody to provide capital for them. I think hospitals and other organizations that are interested in competitively and aggressively moving into health care marketplaces may see the logic in providing the thing that has never been there. This could be the spark that will make group practice explode as it has not done in the past, despite the many who have predicted from time to time that it would.

DR. ELLWOOD: It seems to me that the thing that will cause the scenario that Dr. Nelson described *not* to take place is the tendency for payers to lump multiple providers together.

The groups have been doing very well lately because, while groups typically had high overhead rates and so forth, when you lump them together with efficient use of hospitals, then they suddenly become a much more attractive entity to third parties.

I don't think that the health boutiques are going to successfully operate as independent entities. They're going to be tied in to larger entities because the third-party payers want to make sure that every element of health care the people are using is economically provided and coordinated.

5

The Structure of Hospital-Physician Relationships: The Interplay of Law and Policy

CLARK C. HAVIGHURST

New economic pressures are widely regarded as heralding substantial changes in hospitals' relationships with physicians. One informed observer has recently speculated that the emerging need for effective cost control will force hospitals and their physicians either to integrate more closely (through joint ventures of various kinds) or to draw further apart, dealing with each other more as business adversaries than has been customary under prevailing organizational structures. Already, tendencies in both of these directions can be observed. On the one hand, hospital and physician services have been extensively integrated in health maintenance organizations, and interest in new types of hospital-physician joint ventures is reported to be high. On the other hand, hospitals and physicians are increasingly finding themselves in direct competition with each other in the provision of some ambulatory services. Even where hospital-physician relationships still take their traditional form, new frictions are appearing as hospitals increasingly assert interests at variance with those of their organized medical staffs.

There may be important legal as well as economic reasons for hospital-physician relationships to be either closer or more distant than has been customary. In particular, where the traditional hospital structure featuring an independent, self-governing medical staff is adhered to, a sound reading of antitrust law requires a clearer separation of roles and more independence for the hospital in decision making on questions of staffing. On the other hand, where closer integration is achieved through the formation of a

---

The author is preparing a fuller, documented version of this paper for later publication in the *Duke Law Journal*.

true joint venture, an entirely different legal analysis would apply; thus, if the joint venture itself would pass muster as a pro-competitive undertaking, antitrust law should have nothing to say about its internal structure or decision-making process. If the legal analysis offered here is correct, the law would serve to push hospital-physician relationships in the same directions as efficiency considerations—either toward closer integration or toward true arm's length bargaining by independent business entities. These incentives for reform would appear to be desirable results and thus to be an argument in favor of the legal interpretations offered.

Before addressing the antitrust issues, it is appropriate to comment on the various influences that have shaped hospitals and brought them to the point from which new departures are now proceeding. This discussion will permit some suggestions for changing the legal environment in order not to foreclose hospitals' adaptation to their new economic circumstances.

I. The Expanding Decision-Making Role of Hospitals

The pressures and incentives that are currently changing the environment of hospital decision making are not hard to identify. First, hospitals have new financial problems due to changes in the ways in which they are paid. The most important development is the phase out of retrospective cost reimbursement under the Medicare program and its replacement by DRG allowances. In addition, however, other payers, both public and private, are beginning to negotiate with hospitals and to steer their beneficiaries toward lower cost facilities. Price competition among hospitals is thus gradually becoming a reality. The result of these measures is that hospitals are becoming more cost conscious and are beginning to insist that physicians take account of economic realities in their use of the hospital. Organized medical staffs increasingly perceive their own interest in helping their hospitals to make ends meet and to compete successfully.

A second factor affecting hospital-physician relationships is the recent growth of the physician supply. Hospitals have always needed doctors. For the first time, however, they are now able to acquire them in something other than a seller's market, with the result that a doctor's willingness to cooperate in helping the hospital to solve its cost problem is becoming a factor in the award of admitting privileges. Doctors are being asked to assist in cost containment both through staff committee work and by modifying their styles of practice.

Another aspect of the increased physician supply is the increased threat of litigation when admitting privileges are denied. Not only are denials more frequent, but litigation is more likely because physicians who lose privileges are apt to find it harder to establish themselves elsewhere. Physicians denied privileges may have more reason than previously to suspect anticompetitive motives on the part of their peers in excluding them, and the new availability of antitrust theories, which offer the potential for treble damages if such motives can be proved, makes lawsuits more inviting. Because litigation is costly even if the hospital ultimately prevails, a new seriousness surrounds decisions on staff privileges.

Although these recent changes in the environment of hospitals have increased the interest that hospital boards and administrators take in patient care and in the other activities of doctors in the hospital, the trend in this direction is not really a new thing. A number of earlier developments had very similar effects and produced conflicts similar to, though perhaps not as intense as, those that are being seen today. Notable among these earlier developments are the changes in tort doctrine in the fifties and sixties that significantly increased the exposure of hospitals to personal injury suits. The first of these legal developments, the elimination of charitable immunity, was quickly followed by major changes in doctrines of vicarious liability, which made hospitals responsible, first, for the negligence of their professional employees and, later, for the work of professionals who, while not technically employees, were perceived by patients to be agents of the hospital. In particular, the famous *Darling* case in Illinois in 1965 imposed liability on a hospital for an injury caused by an attending physician assigned to duty in the emergency room; much more surprising than the legal result in that case was the widespread reaction to it, which suggested that hospital managers had been waiting for some excuse to assert themselves in demanding more cooperation from their medical staffs. Finally, since the *Darling* case, a number of decisions have held hospitals negligent for not screening their professional staff more carefully. Although the cumulative effect of all these changes in tort law was a strengthening of hospitals' stake in the quality of care being provided, it is widely believed that many hospitals still do not take enough care to ensure that physicians using the facility actively police each other in the interest of the institution.

Another earlier source of conflict between hospitals and doctors was the growth of cost-containment regulation in the seventies. Much of such regulation focused on the hospital, in part because it represented the "big ticket" item in the overall health care budget, but also because the hospital offered an organizational nexus through which pressure could be brought to bear on physicians and physician behavior could be changed. Certificate-of-need laws were seen as a way of curbing the effects of unbridled hospital competition for doctors and of making it easier for hospital administrators to say no to physicians' demands for more and better facilities. Such laws were also conceived as a way of limiting the resources available to doctors, thus forcing them to ration care. State rate setting programs, limiting hospital revenues, were favored for similar reasons. Indeed, the DRG payment system is only the latest in a series of efforts to get at doctors by imposing economic constraints on hospitals. Over time, as these external constraints have intensified, hospitals have become less and less pliable in their dealings with physicians.

Yet another development that has changed the tone and character of hospital-physician relations has been the expanded role of investor-owned hospitals. These institutions are generally more inclined than their nonprofit counterparts to insist on their own interests in dealing with physicians. Although all hospitals have become more businesslike in recent years, the example of the proprietaries and the competition they provide to the nonprofits have undoubtedly had something to do with this development. In general, it is likely that physicians are finding hospitals to be more like traditional business enterprises and less like private clubs than they used to be.

II. The Balance of Power in Hospitals

Hospitals have acquired the powers they need to discharge their expanding responsibilities for both the quality and the cost of hospital care largely at the expense of physicians. It is thus natural to ask whether the balance of power in hospitals is now roughly correct or whether, by some standard, one or the other party exercises undue influence. Not only is this question probably unanswerable as an abstract proposition, however; it is also not a particularly helpful way to formulate or approach the ultimate policy issues. Sound policy, I submit, would leave the appropriate balance of power in a hospital to be determined in each institution under the constraints that are imposed by external pressures and circumstances. If problems exist, and they do, it is very likely that their true source lies elsewhere than in the hospital itself.

Economists who study and seek to predict hospital behavior have long been interested in what they call hospitals' "objective function": What goals do they pursue? What do they seek to maximize—the corporation's profits, its budget, its rate of growth; the perquisites, prestige, and job security of management; the health of the community; or something else? Some analyses of these questions have concluded that hospital behavior can best be predicted by assuming that physicians are in control. Although such a conclusion might be viewed as proof of some kind of conspiracy, it does not necessarily establish that the influence of physicians over hospitals is a problem to be remedied by some specific intervention. Whereas conspiracy may have strengthened the power of physicians over the operation of hospitals in the past, changes in the market and legal environment may already be undermining the conditions that made such physician dominance possible.

The obvious benefits that physicians derive from their association with hospitals do not, in themselves, prove the existence of any problems originating within the hospital itself. The things that lead economists to find that physicians dominate hospital decision making may be simply artifacts of other problems in the health care marketplace whose removal—if they could be attacked directly—would bring about appropriate adjustments in hospital behavior. Until recently, for example, hospitals had to satisfy their need for physicians in a market with a short supply; it should therefore be no surprise that physicians benefitted in their bargaining with hospitals. Similarly, because third-party financing has made it unnecessary for either hospitals or physicians to count costs closely, there has been little reason for hospitals not to gratify doctors' expensive wishes. Finally, because physicians seeking hospital privileges act in important respects as agents of their insured patients, who also are interested in high-quality care, what appear to be physician gains in bargaining with hospitals may also represent benefits to consumers.

For these reasons, it cannot be concluded that the hospital is itself a significant source of the health care system's difficulties in efficiently allocating societal resources. Of course, if effective competition is lacking or constrained in the markets where hospitals and physicians get together, one may reasonably doubt that bargaining between them is yielding appropriate outcomes and relationships. More important, however, the existence of competition in such markets is far from a sufficient condition for efficiency. Indeed, even if we could directly intervene in hospitals and solve any problems that we find there, we would still have made little progress toward curing the larger problems of distorted incentives and weak price competition that are the product of dysfunctional financing mechanisms. By the same token, however, attention to these latter problems would probably go rather far toward stimulating needed changes in the operation of hospitals and in hospital-doctor relations. As noted earlier, the important changes and power shifts that are currently occurring in hospitals are direct reflections of external forces that are increasingly impinging on health care providers.

III. The Internal Organization of Hospitals

Despite the overriding importance of the external environment in shaping power relationships within hospitals, a look inside the hospital reveals some problems that may not yield readily to outside pressures and market forces. M.I.T. economist Jeffrey Harris has observed that there is an almost complete separation in hospitals of what he calls the "revenue centers," which physicians control, from the "cost centers," which are the province of administrators. Harris notes that the institutionalized barriers he perceives between those whose decisions generate demands on the hospital and those who must provide the resources to meet those demands create severe difficulties for hospitals in controlling their costs. The separation of hospital and physician decision makers is strongly reinforced by the existence of an independent, self-governing medical staff and by the convention of billing patients separately for hospital and physician services.

It is paradoxical that the sharp separation of operational responsibilities within hospitals results in some measure from a closeness in policy making between the typical hospital governing board and the medical staff. It is widely suspected that many hospital boards, particularly in nonprofit institutions, while they retain formal power, have effectively yielded most of their decision-making authority on a wide range of issues to the medical staff.

If it is true that hospitals defer to physicians and seldom actively assert their independent, and sometimes conflicting, interests, it would follow that hospitals' internal structures and operations excessively reflect the preferences of physicians. On the other hand, as hospitals face increasing cost pressures, they are likely to begin to reclaim some of their lost or shared authority, thus distancing themselves from physicians in the decision-making process. They may also then proceed to reorganize themselves in more efficient ways, perhaps breaking down the extreme separation of functions that Harris observes. Whether public policymakers need to focus any special attention on hospitals' decision-making mechanisms or organizational structures depends on whether hospitals face any artificial constraints in reshaping themselves to realize their corporate purposes. An answer to this latter question may perhaps be found by inquiring further into why hospitals are organized as they are.

Though Harris notes that one could attribute the extreme separation of responsibilities in hospitals to a desire "to perpetuate an organized medical monopoly," he sees a more benign explanation. Adopting a perspective very similar to that taken by economist Kenneth Arrow in a well-known 1963 article, Harris attributes the hospital's internal structure to the special nature of medical care, particularly the ethical dimension of the doctor-patient relationship and the need, particularly in hospitals, to cope rapidly with complexity and uncertainty without pausing to calculate benefit-cost ratios. Harris's interpretation seems to owe much to the fact that he is trained in medicine as well as economics. However, it is not clear whether this unusual perspective enables him to see values that escape more cynical observers or instead makes him less inclined to question the motives that led hospitals to be organized in a way that causes systematic neglect of the cost factor. In any event, Harris never clearly asks why it was that internal hospital arrangements such as those that he himself proposes as reforms never evolved of their own accord.

Harris's attribution of the prevailing organizational pattern in hospitals to patient care considerations seems subject to much the same criticism that sociologist Paul Starr has offered of Arrow's earlier profession of admiration for the systematically anticompetitive institutional arrangements that he identified in medical care. Arrow, says Starr, writes "as if some inner dynamic were pushing the world toward Pareto optimality." Finding in Arrow a "presumption that what is real is rational or, as the economists say, 'optimal,'" Starr concludes that the result of Arrow's analysis "is not so much to explain as to explain away the particular institutional structure medical care has assumed in the United States." Harris, though noting the need for organizational changes in hospitals, was similarly uncritical of the process by which hospitals came to be organized as they are. In short, neither Arrow nor Harris adequately recognizes that the financing and organizational arrangements they contemplated were designed in large part by organized medicine. In each case, it seems probable that a major goal of dominant professional interests in designing institutional frameworks was to remove physicians as far as possible from cost and competitive pressures.

In the case of hospitals, the organizational characteristics noted by Harris are not the result of considered choices by hospital managers about how best to organize and operate a hospital. Nor is the reason why nearly all hospitals are organized in essentially the same fashion to be found in the operation of the marketplace's invisible hand. Instead, it appears that hospitals' internal structures have been prescribed by the Joint Commission on the Accreditation of Hospitals (JCAH), a body dominated by representatives of powerful medical organizations. In addition to mandating the existence of an independent, self-governing medical staff, JCAH accreditation standards contemplate essentially the same departmental configuration that Harris finds inefficient for the task of cost containment. Although this internal structure probably could not have been imposed on hospitals if external conditions had been substantially different, the medical profession apparently exercised enough control over the payment system and the physician supply to permit physicians to obtain hospital privileges on their desired terms. It should not be surprising if we find that, as designed by the JCAH, hospitals unduly serve the interests of physicians.

Legal requirements, though important, do not appear to have been the dominant factor determining the internal organization of hospitals. Statutes that today require hospitals in some states to maintain a self-governing medical staff appear to have been enacted only after that model became dominant, perhaps because professional interests were concerned about deviations from this norm by smaller, unaccredited institutions. Perhaps the most important legal influences in the early days were legal rules restricting in varying degrees the corporate practice of medicine. Nevertheless, although these rules barred many hospitals from providing professional services to patients through their own employees, they did not make it inevitable that lay hospital boards would create a self-governing medical staff and delegate to it responsibility for all medical matters. There were other organizational arrangements, between directly employing physicians and relying upon an independent medical staff, that hospitals could have lawfully adopted to carry out their corporate purposes. For example, a hospital might have integrated its cost and revenue centers, might have hired physicians to administer its operating units, and might have contracted directly with individual physicians desiring to use the facility. Instead of relying on an independent medical component to provide peer review, a hospital might have empowered its own physician-administrators to oversee a physician's practice in the interest of quality assurance and cost containment. The almost universal neglect of such alternatives for lawfully and efficiently organizing a hospital without an independent medical staff strongly suggests that the medical profession, working largely through the JCAH in recent years, has effectively controlled the terms upon which hospitals may deal with physicians.

Although the JCAH has been effective in protecting physician interests in the past, it may be less so in the future. Already it has been compelled by fear of antitrust action to change one of its most cherished standards—that which flatly excluded nonphysician providers from eligibility for admitting privileges. The JCAH future influence may also be reduced as a result of recent antitrust scholarship pointing out flaws in its constitution. Whatever may happen on the antitrust front, the changing economic environment could induce an increasing number of hospitals to design their future arrangements with doctors without regard to JCAH requirements. Thus, a hospital might decide to rewrite its medical staff's bylaws without the staff's consent, even though that act would jeopardize the hospital's accreditation. Another hospital, facing financial difficulties and the loss of accreditation for quality deficiencies, might elect to adopt organizational reforms of which it knows the JCAH will disapprove. In short, growing economic pressures, coupled with changes in the JCAH itself, could eventually inspire a significant number of hospitals to alter those arrangements mandated by the JCAH that have heretofore insulated individual physicians from direct accountability to the hospital.

The possibility that hospital decision making is unduly dominated by physicians is a policy problem that cuts across the entire spectrum of hospital behavior, triggering major concerns about whether resources are being allocated to their best uses. Although solutions to the overall resource allocation problem must be pursued primarily through incentive-oriented reforms and not within the hospital itself, such reforms should be accompanied by careful attention to any legal, regulatory, and extralegal constraints that may inhibit the changes that must occur inside the hospitals before consumer preferences can be effectively translated into provider behavior. The legal system currently influences hospital-physician relationships and the internal organization of hospitals in several ways. The remainder of this paper highlights some of these influences and suggests some legal changes or reinterpretations that would allow hospital-physician relationships to evolve in desirable ways under the overall influence of market forces. Although what follows is not a legal treatise, it is intended to clarify the implications of legal doctrine for the smooth functioning of the health care marketplace. As the health care industry comes to be seen as a province in which market forces can be constructive instruments of social control and resource allocation, courts and legal analysts must reexamine old premises in a new light. It goes almost without saying that statutes directly regulating hospitals' arrangements with physicians and judge-made rules restricting the corporate practice of medicine and the direct employment of physicians may no longer be appropriate limitations on hospitals' freedom to organize themselves to meet the challenges that they are being asked to meet.

IV. The Hospital Medical Staff and the Law— An Antitrust Perspective

Aside from those statutes and rules that directly regulate hospitals' internal organization, most of the law governing the hospital medical staff involves the award or denial of hospital admitting privileges. Because a medical staff is a combination of competing physicians, however, it is subject in all of its activities to legal scrutiny under section 1 of the Sherman Act. Thus, although staff privileges are the main topic of discussion here, it is important at the outset to understand the antitrust rationale under which a medical staff is permitted to exist and the substantial limitations that rationale places on the staff's activities and methods of operation.

A. THE MEDICAL STAFF AS A PROCOMPETITIVE
COLLABORATION OF COMPETING PHYSICIANS

A hospital medical staff is organized at the invitation of a hospital, which looks to it to perform a variety of services vital to the hospital's overall health care mission. As one element in an enterprise that must compete with other comparable enterprises, the staff serves a clear procompetitive purpose and is therefore presumptively entitled to have any anticompetitive effects judged under the antitrust laws as so-called ancillary restraints—that is, as incidental restraints necessary to the accomplishment of a legitimate business purpose. Thus, if the staff's organization and activities are reasonably well tailored to accomplish legitimate hospital objectives, no antitrust objection should ordinarily be raised. For example, staff-imposed limitations on members' surgical privileges, though technically a division of markets, could be justified by reference to the hospital's competitive incentive (not to mention its legal duty) to ensure that its surgeons are competent to perform the tasks they undertake. Other staff activities related to quality assurance and cost containment would also be defensible by reference to the hospital's business and competitive interests. It is notable that such self-policing activities are not upheld because they are in some sense "in the public interest" or because they are undertaken by professionals rather than ordinary mortals. Antitrust law does not, as a general rule, permit competitor collaboration simply because it serves worthy purposes, professional or otherwise, but focuses instead on whether a particular collaboration is compatible with the maintenance of competition in the market as a whole. It is nevertheless usually the case, as here, that activities deemed to be procompetitive are desirable in other respects.

The requirement that a hospital medical staff must be able to justify its anticompetitive activities by reference to the hospital's purposes has an important corollary—namely that the staff may not rely on purposes of its own to justify an anticompetitive action. Thus, there is no warrant in standard antitrust doctrine for a medical staff's acting as a unit for collective bargaining. Although there would be no objection to the staff's collective advocacy of policies that the hospital board might adopt, the line of illegality is crossed if physicians should take or threaten to take concerted action against the hospital—such as taking their patients elsewhere—if their collective wishes are not granted.

There is little doubt that independent physicians are not free—as employees organized into a labor union are free, for example—to make collective decisions about whether, when, where, or on what terms to supply their services. It is of course often difficult to distinguish between a threat to take collective action and a mere prediction that individuals will act in a certain way in certain circumstances, but the law is quite clear in prohibiting naked group boycotts and concerted refusals to deal. Though many medical staffs probably violate this basic rule frequently in their dealings with hospitals, few are likely to be caught. However, five doctors in a Texas town were recently sued successfully by the FTC for attempting to dictate a hospital's decisions. Physicians should be advised that their financial liability could be substantial if they should carry out their threat to harm the hospital or if a plaintiff could prove that he lost business or employment as a result of their pressure on the hospital.

An implication of the antitrust rule under which medical staff actions are tested by reference to the hospital's business purposes is that the staff is a subsidiary and not an independent element within the hospital and is subject in the last analysis to the authority of the governing board. This view is essentially consistent both with basic concepts of corporation law and with the view of the hospital-staff relationship that is set forth in JCAH standards. Although it should not be controversial, some attempts to pursue the implications of this formal structure may be found so. It is argued below that antitrust courts should be specifically concerned in each case with whether the hospital board maintained its independence or instead joined a physician conspiracy by abdicating its formal responsibilities.

B. THE COMMON LAW OF HOSPITAL STAFF PRIVILEGES—THE NEED FOR A NEW RATIONALE

It is widely remarked that the law governing the award of hospital admitting privileges forces hospitals to steer a treacherous course. On the one hand, the Scylla of tort law imposes on hospitals a duty to exercise due care in deciding which providers can use their facilities. On the other hand, a Charybdis of common-law doctrines, statutory rules, and antitrust principles threatens a hospital with substantial burdens and penalties if it should act unfairly or illegally in denying, revoking, or curtailing an individual provider's privileges. Rather than undertaking a full treatment of all of these subjects, this paper concentrates on conceptualizing the antitrust principles applicable to current practices in awarding hospital staff privileges. Because this analysis focuses attention on the dynamic features of hospital-physician relationships, the allocation of decision-making responsibility, and the overriding interest of consumers, it should be helpful to courts that are asked to review denials of staff privileges under common-law principles.

Common-law courts in a number of jurisdictions have conferred substantial legal protections upon applicants for hospital admitting privileges, mostly by being prepared to review hospital actions under norms of substantive and procedural due process. Though well established, these fairness requirements, which are applicable in some degree to private as well as public hospitals, appear to need rethinking in the light of recent developments in national health policy and the evolution of the health care industry toward organization and operation along more competitive lines. When active enforcement of the antitrust laws against health care providers began in the late seventies, there occurred, almost ipso facto, a redefinition of national policy toward the health care sector. In effect, the antitrust initiative reversed a federal policy of tacitly accepting the prevalent view among health care providers that they were justified in insulating themselves from competitive pressures. Whereas doubts about the value and appropriateness of competition in health care had previously weakened the resolve of courts and enforcement agencies to insist upon competition, leaving policy in a kind of limbo, federal policy today rather clearly starts from the proposition that the health care sector is a competitive industry to be guided by market forces, for better or for worse, unless Congress expressly declares otherwise or unless regulatory controls are clearly substituted.

The common-law courts that came to oversee hospitals' denials of privileges did so in an environment substantially different from the current one. Moreover, they expressly found their authority in a conception of the hospital as a quasi-public enterprise or public utility rather than as a private business operating in an essentially competitive environment. It is far from clear today why hospitals are under any greater obligations than typical employers to account to the courts for the fairness with which they screen applicants for professional positions or why health care professionals deserve any special legal help in surmounting marketplace barriers to their pursuit of their livelihoods. The due process requirements which common-law courts have required hospitals to observe in denying staff privileges are in fact anomalous and find weak support in the common-law ground in which they are rooted.

A reexamination of the staff privileges issue in light of the new economic environment and more market-oriented national policies toward the health care sector would suggest that common-law courts, instead of applying to hospitals norms drawn from constitutional or public utility law, should ground their review of privileges decisions in tort principles applicable to unfair competition. This approach would call appropriate attention to the frequently controlling influence of physician competitors of an applicant for privileges. Adoption of the unfair competition rationale would also, like the antitrust analysis below, ensure that any decision that was made by and in the interest of the hospital itself and not by the medical staff alone would be permitted to stand unless contrary to statutory law. Moreover, judicial review of medical staff activities under such a tort rationale would not simply duplicate antitrust remedies. Not only would a tort action not require proof of an effect on interstate commerce, but it would focus substantially more on issues of fairness than would an antitrust court, which should be primarily concerned with the protection of "competition, not competitors." Despite the somewhat different emphasis of antitrust law, the antitrust discussion that follows should significantly assist common-law courts in dealing with the complicated and hotly disputed factual situations they confront in privilege cases.

C. AN APPLICATION OF ANTITRUST PRINCIPLES TO DECISIONS ON HOSPITAL ADMITTING PRIVILEGES

Antitrust analysis of privileges issues have not yet succeeded in clarifying the law, simplifying its application, or giving hospitals and their medical staffs clear guidance so that they can pursue the institution's competitive goals in reasonable safety. The most thorough and thoughtful examination of the privileges problem, that of Phillip Kissam et al. ("Antitrust and Hospital Privileges," *California Law Review* 70 [May 1982]: 595–685), recommends that the courts, in most cases, should seek to discover whether the "predominant purpose" served by a denial of privileges was an anticompetitive one, and similar views have been adopted in the few district court decisions that have dealt with privileges denials on the merits. This purpose-oriented approach is unsatisfactory, however, because it offers few short cuts by which courts can avoid a lengthy trial of strongly contested factual issues. The legal rationale sketched here is primarily an attempt to isolate some key factors by which easy cases can be quickly resolved in hospitals' favor, thereby reducing litigation fears that may hamper efforts to achieve efficiency and improve the quality of care. Although not exhaustive in its legal analysis, the discussion shows how clarity could be achieved and how the law could be made compatible with overriding policy objectives.

1. *Avoiding hospital involvement in a physician conspiracy.* In dealing with its medical staff, a hospital must be careful not to be drawn into a doctor conspiracy. Certainly a hospital is not guilty of an antitrust violation simply because it sets up an independent medical staff and enters into agreements or understandings with it; there are good business reasons for its doing so—if only to earn JCAH accreditation. But a failure to oversee and control the medical staff could properly be deemed to involve the hospital as an equal partner in any anticompetitive action taken by the staff in the hospital's name. An antitrust court would be justified in closely scrutinizing the actions of this larger combination. It is argued here that judicial scrutiny in such a case should be more searching than in a case where the hospital acted independently in its own interest, thus serving as a check on the staff's power.

Courts have so far not recognized the central importance of the hospital's decision-making independence in antitrust cases involving admitting privileges. Although in some cases the hospital's governing board plainly acted independently, courts have not regarded that fact as calling for any different legal test than would be applied if the actual decision makers were physician competitors of the plaintiff. Nevertheless, the significance of this issue for antitrust purposes can be established by applying the general principle of antitrust analysis which holds that a procompetitive purpose cannot justify an incidental restriction on competition if that same purpose could have been achieved by some less restrictive means. Although this principle has not been made a firm legal requirement and would do harm if it were applied so rigorously as to make the best always the enemy of the good, it appears to be helpful in defining the type of relationship that hospitals must maintain with their physicians. If competition is seriously endangered by the hospital's creation of a self-governing medical staff, an antitrust court might reasonably expect the hospital to maintain, as a "less restrictive alternative," an independent check on the staff's activities. Such a requirement would help to ensure that the medical staff's collective decisions do not become hospital policy unless the hospital governing board, acting independently, concurs for reasons of its own.

Many actions of a medical staff with respect to staffing and personnel policy do indeed carry a potential for anticompetitive abuse. Individual physicians applying for admitting privileges may be turned down because staff physicians wish to retain the competitive advantage of access to the hospital's possibly unique facilities. Likewise, formal prerequisites for admitting privileges, such as a requirement for specialty board certification or for malpractice insurance coverage, might be established primarily to exclude low-priced competitors. Similarly, a hospital's policy on the admission of patients under the care of nonphysician providers might easily reflect staff physicians' fear of competition over both price and ideology. Finally, decisions to close the staff to new applicants, while possibly indicated by operational and quality considerations, might also be inspired by desire of the "haves" on the medical staff to exclude the "have nots." Because anticompetitive motives may easily influence the medical staff's judgment on all such matters, antitrust courts should see a real need for the hospital to act independently.

An antitrust court could greatly reduce the potential for anticompetitive abuse of the medical staff's power by increasing the depth of judicial inquiry—and thus the hospital's exposure to liability—whenever it examines a decision that was dominated by staff physicians. By the same token, courts should be more easily persuaded to grant summary judgment or a directed verdict in a hospital's favor whenever a plaintiff cannot demonstrate that the decision being challenged was something other than a hospital business decision. Under the legal test proposed here, a hospital would be able to protect itself by showing from its internal documents that it was free to consult its own interests in making the decision and was not bound to any extent by any action of the staff. It should also be clear from board minutes and otherwise that the board did in fact act independently on the issue in question and did consider the hospital's interests, including its interest in attracting the patients of the excluded provider. Finally, the hospital's case would be further strengthened if it appeared that the board recognized the staff's conflict of interests and made some effort to satisfy itself concerning the strength of the evidence supporting the staff's recommendation. For example, an independent appraisal of an individual using outside professional evaluators would, in addition to being sound management, demonstrate that the board's objective was not to satisfy the medical staff but to serve institutional goals. Having made a proper record, showing diligent performance of its corporate responsibilities, a hospital should be able to obtain summary judgment in many cases, perhaps even before extensive discovery was ordered.

2. *The appropriate degree and nature of judicial scrutiny.* The goal of facilitating early dismissal of antitrust cases that challenge staffing decisions by hospital boards acting independently can be achieved only if such decisions are subject to a degree of judicial scrutiny that can be exercised without exhaustive discovery or a full trial. The proper test would appear to be a rational-basis test under which the decision would be upheld upon the discovery of any plausible basis related to a legitimate interest of the hospital. Thus, summary judgment or a directed verdict would be appropriate in any case where the hospital's decision seemed plausibly related to its natural concerns about its reputation, the quality of care offered, its exposure to malpractice suits, its efficient and profitable operation, or the maintenance of harmonious relationships within the institution.

Some courts would be naturally inclined to scrutinize a hospital's judgment more closely to see whether the ostensible reasons were its real reasons or whether the decision's adverse effect on competition among providers was justified by its actual contribution to fulfilling the hospital's objectives. Nevertheless, that approach would amount to a misuse of the less-restrictive-alternative requirement, converting it from a simple reasonableness test into a warrant for closely regulating private procompetitive behavior. Courts should strongly resist the temptation to verify that each specific action had a net procompetitive effect. Instead, they should employ the antitrust rule of reason to ensure that arrangements are structured in ways that do not belie their ostensible purposes and that seem likely to enhance competition and promote efficiency.

The hardest cases for courts to dismiss summarily will be those in which a decision by a hospital board in concurrence with the medical staff, in addition to arguably improving the competitive effectiveness of the institution, also advances other, less laudable interests of the hospital. One category of such cases would be those in which the hospital, instead of (or in addition to) serving the anticompetitive interests of its physicians, appeared to have anticompetitive interests of its own. The best example would be a hospital which, with debatable reasons, refused admitting privileges to physicians associated with a fledgling HMO, perhaps in the hope that the HMO would disappear if its access to the hospital were limited. Though having no hospital of its own, an HMO is properly viewed as a competitor of the hospital itself because it frequently substitutes outpatient for inpatient services; moreover, the HMO may be feared because it is likely to become a hard, price-conscious bargainer with the hospital. Although it may be difficult to determine whether the hospital acted on its own or made common cause with its medical staff, the existence of a hospital-physician conspiracy would not be a prerequisite to obtaining antitrust relief in such circumstances. The hospital's conduct—a refusal to deal with physicians who associate with its competitor—might be scrutinized as a unilateral attempt to monopolize. Or, if such a theory is not available because the presence of other hospitals in the community belies the requisite dangerous probability of monopoly, a successful conspiracy case might be built against the several hospitals if they all refused to compete for the HMO's paying patients. In any event, an antitrust solution to the problem of anti-HMO conduct by a hospital does not require finding a hospital-physician conspiracy and can be pursued without violating the principles suggested here.

Another category of cases in which a court might be induced to subject a hospital's independent conduct to close rather than limited scrutiny would be those in which a hospital could be suspected of acting as the doctors' "cat's paw" in suppressing competition that they find objectionable. Governing board members might, for example, hold the view that the hospital's long-run interest is best served by going along with the medical staff in borderline cases even at some cost to the hospital itself. Indeed, in a given case, a hospital decision to exclude nonphysician practitioners or to classify a doctor's personality as disruptive might be a response, not to the hospital's perception of its own competitive situation, but to a collective threat by doctors to retaliate in some fashion if the hospital should pursue its own interests. In such circumstances, although the case for finding a conspiracy with physicians would be strong, the question would remain whether close scrutiny—that is, a full inquiry into all of the surrounding circumstances—should be employed to ascertain the predominant motive underlying the hospital's decision or the net effect of its action on consumer welfare. Instead of adopting this approach, a court might elect—because the hospital board acted independently—still to engage in only limited scrutiny, seeking only some plausible relation between the hospital's action and a legitimate procompetitive purpose. Unless this latter view is taken, most hospital decisions that happen to advance the interests of the medical staff would be subject to close scrutiny. Indeed, the analyses in the Kissam article and the recent cases seem to proceed as if the merest possibility of a hospital-physician conspiracy must always trigger a full investigation.

It is problematical whether courts can be persuaded to exercise restraint in reviewing hospital decisions which, though independent, suggest possible involvement in a physician conspiracy. Antitrust courts have long demonstrated an excessive propensity for closely examining the conduct of a single firm whenever it affects competition in another market. This propensity is most pronounced in the law relating to so-called vertical restraints—that is, to restrictions placed by a manufacturer on competition in the distribution of his products. Because this is a controversial area of the law at the moment, recognizing any analogy between hospitals' staffing decisions and vertical restraints may be counterproductive in the effort to achieve legal clarity. Nevertheless, the current trend in the law of vertical restraints is to recognize the overriding importance of competition among manufacturers—"interbrand" as opposed to "intrabrand" competition—and to accord some deference to a manufacturer's efforts to structure an efficient distribution system through which to compete with other manufacturers. Although vertical restraints still appear to be subject to condemnation if they seem, under close scrutiny, to reflect a manufacturer's participation in a horizontal conspiracy of its distributors, the hospital-physician case seems significantly different because of the close relationship that must exist between a hospital and its medical staff. As discussed further below, the degree of integration inside a hospital, while not complete enough to insulate hospital-physician relationships from even limited antitrust scrutiny, should be deemed sufficient to spare a responsible hospital the burden of close scrutiny.

Thus, close scrutiny by antitrust courts of hospital actions that serve the competitive interests of the medical staff seems appropriately reserved for those cases in which the hospital appears to have acted, not as an independent decision maker, but as a rubber stamp for its doctors' decision. On the face of it, it would seem wrong to impose the same burden of proof and risk of liability on an institution that had acted affirmatively to minimize the danger of anticompetitive abuse by the medical staff by interposing a responsible hospital board as an independent check on the doctors' power; it would be very hard doctrine indeed, especially given the JCAH requirement, to say that the hospital had a less restrictive alternative to maintaining an organized medical staff and must therefore accept close scrutiny by courts seeking to avert hazards that it voluntarily created. By the same token, individual physicians participating in the useful work of a medical staff ought not to be exposed to an undue risk of suits by individuals who are injured and offended by their honest efforts; a rule distinguishing between hospital actions and actions effectively controlled by the medical staff would go far toward protecting the physicians involved so long as they submit fully to the authority of the hospital board.

The legal rule suggested here calls attention to a structural problem within hospitals that courts have heretofore generally ignored. If adopted, it would inspire hospitals to assume decision making responsibilities that are legally and rightfully theirs but which some hospital boards, particularly in nonprofit institutions, have passively allowed to devolve on medical staffs without appreciable accountability. By strengthening the hand and the backbone of hospitals vis-á-vis their physicians, the suggested rule would contribute to the achievement of the policy goal of helping hospitals respond appropriately to their changing economic environment. On the other hand, a rule subjecting all hospitals to severe litigation risks regardless of whether they had acted to minimize the influence of physicians over particular decisions would unduly inhibit hospital efforts to ensure the competence of physicians and to obtain their cooperation in the cost-containment effort. Under such a rule, the liability risks and litigation expenses faced by hospitals and physicians, the costs of which undoubtedly exceed any reasonable measure of the harm to the public in a given case, would create an excessive incentive for hospitals to resolve close questions in favor of providers whose performance is in doubt. Thus, if judges undertake to search out and, if necessary, rectify unfairness to competitors, they are likely to reduce consumer welfare.

The danger presented here is thus a fundamental and recurring one in antitrust law—namely that courts, asked to ensure that a particular plaintiff was fairly treated and mistakenly believing that protecting competitors is the same thing as protecting competition, will penalize the selectivity that is vital to the achievement of efficiency in free markets. It is believed that the analysis here strikes the right balance between fairness and efficiency concerns by stressing the importance of ascertaining that decisions are made by the parties most likely to act for the benefit of consumers and by protecting those decision makers, and those whom they commission to advise them, from litigation risks that can only diminish their efforts to serve consumers well.

3. *Antitrust rules in action.* The effect of a rule extending a high degree of deference to staffing decisions when they appear truly to be decisions of the hospital itself and not decisions of the medical staff can be appreciated more fully by considering a hypothetical case. Assume that Dr. X has had his privileges at each of the three hospitals in his community revoked because of his allegedly disruptive personality. Cases of this kind are not uncommon and appear to present some troublesome possibilities. It is the task of courts to uncover the abuses without preempting or inhibiting legitimate private decision making.

The first question is whether Dr. X can make a legal case against any of the hospitals. Under the rule proposed above, the court should be satisfied if the hospital made an independent decision on plausible grounds to terminate Dr. X. The following questions would be relevant to the decision whether to grant either summary judgment on the basis of documentary evidence or a directed verdict following plaintiff's initial effort to prove a hospital-physician conspiracy:

Did the hospital's decision-making process demonstrate its independence?

Did the board consider the possibility of bias on the part of the staff decision makers and do anything to ensure that it was getting sound advice?

Did the medical staff offer good professional reasons of a kind that the hospital might regard as valid?

Did the hospital board seek to verify these reasons? Did it, for example, seek outside advice or make inquiry of key witnesses under circumstances ensuring that their testimony was not coerced?

Did the board consider any countervailing factors? For example, if Dr. X's patients brought a quarter million dollars to the hospital each year, did the hospital board consider that fact?

Does it appear from the record, or was it plausible, that Dr. X was judged by the board to be enough of a problem to warrant giving up the revenue he represented? Lest it be thought that a crass trade-off between profits and quality would be unseemly, it should be observed that the money generated by Dr. X could be used to improve the quality of the hospital in other ways.

Only if the hospital's independence of judgment and action does not appear on the face of the record should a hospital-physician conspiracy (or combination, to use the less pejorative statutory term) be found. In the absence of such a conspiracy, there would be on these facts sufficient business reason for the hospital to terminate Dr. X, and the case should come to an end. On the other hand, if a conspiracy (combination) should appear, the court should proceed to evaluate the underlying motives of the hospital and medical staff, an inquiry that would usually require a full trial unless the medical staff had itself so structured things, through fair procedures and appointment of clearly disinterested decision makers, as to remove the danger of competitor bias. The ultimate question would remain whether, judged in depth, the hospital-physician action was the result of a business decision taken on behalf of the hospital as a competitive enterprise. Although the decided cases have generally approached privilege cases in roughly this fashion, their failure to distinguish between hospital-dominated and physician-dominated decisions may have made them more demanding in some situations and less demanding in others than is warranted by vital antitrust concerns.

In Dr. X's case, it might be thought that the concurrence of the other hospitals supported the result at each institution. Another and more ominous possibility, however, is that there was a community-wide hospital or hospital-physician boycott aimed at Dr. X. This possibility should be taken seriously because some medical communities have been accustomed to operate in just such a way, assuming essentially regulatory power over who can and who cannot practice in the area. Although the existence of a larger conspiracy would probably have to be proved circumstantially, it is quite likely that Dr. X would be able to show, as one element of his proof, that there was a great deal of communication among the members of the respective medical staffs. The inference of conspiracy would be further supported if one or more hospitals had departed from the regular schedule for reviewing Dr. X's status. Unless explained by the egregiousness of Dr. X's sins, this unusual coordination of action would permit a judge or jury to find collusion based on the likelihood that each hospital, fearful of losing the revenue represented by Dr. X, was hesitant to act unless the others did so as well. Antitrust law has well-developed theories for analyzing such "conscious parallelism" and would permit a judge or jury to find a hospital boycott on this evidence.

If such a boycott were found, it should certainly be treated as a per se violation, so that there could be no defense predicated on the notion that eliminating Dr. X was a service to the community. Although a few courts have hesitated to apply the per se rule to true boycotts by health care providers, the situation here would deserve no such leniency. Under basic antitrust precepts, Dr. X is entitled to the benefit of truly independent hospital decisions regarding his qualifications and desirability. Although it can be highly beneficial and procompetitive for competitors to share information and even to offer their opinions concerning their competitors' qualifications, in no event should sellers or buyers acting in concert finally judge competing sellers. In health care markets, hospitals clearly need information and professional help in judging physicians, but the antitrust laws are appropriately invoked to ensure that, in the final analysis, the individual hospitals themselves make the final decisions. The analysis herein seeks to realize this essential value.

V. Hospital-Physician Joint Ventures

It was noted at the outset of this paper that competitive forces and the pursuit of efficiency may require hospitals either to get closer to their physicians or to separate themselves further from them. The antitrust analysis just offered of traditional hospital-physician relationship suggests that there are good legal reasons for hospitals to widen the distance between themselves and their physicians by asserting their independence from the medical staff in making personnel and staffing policy decisions. The discussion here briefly considers the quite different legal analysis that would apply if hospitals and physicians should elect to move in the opposite direction, away from the separate existence implied by the traditional model and toward more integrated arrangements.

In order to compete more effectively in a cost-conscious environment, many hospitals are currently exploring the possibilities for entering into joint ventures with their physicians. Most of the arrangements being considered would involve the creation of a single corporate entity under the joint control of the hospital and the physician group. Under the antitrust laws, the creation of such a joint venture must be scrutinized with care to determine whether competition is being sacrificed. But if the venture survives this analysis, it should be relatively free of the kind of judicial interference that is deemed necessary when independent entities interact without totally integrating their activities.

One reason why it has been predicted that hospital-physician relations will become less friendly and more adversarial in the future is that there are increasing opportunities for each class of provider to enter markets occupied by the other. Partly to increase the flow of patients, hospitals are currently expanding their capacity to provide outpatient services by opening clinics staffed by salaried doctors, thus directly competing for patients with their staff physicians. At the same time, many physicians are offering new services of a kind that have traditionally been provided by hospitals. Thus, physicians have purchased expensive diagnostic equipment for their offices, have sponsored the development of ambulatory surgical facilities, and have opened clinics for the treatment of minor emergencies. To the extent that hospital-physician joint ventures are intended to, or do in fact, have the effect of heading off such competition, they are subject to possible antitrust challenge. The legal tests for appraising their legality require a comparison of the procompetitive benefits of the joint undertaking with the harms to competition that are likely to result. The primary concern is whether there remains in the community a substantial number of other providers offering or capable of offering competitive services. Unfortunately, the tests are necessarily imprecise. However, hospital-physician joint ventures in smaller communities are likely to present severe problems.

If a joint venture is safe from condemnation under the foregoing merger-type analysis, the degree of scrutiny to which its operations and activities will thereafter be subject should depend in part upon the completeness of the integration achieved. Thus, a complete amalgamation of a hospital and physicians into, say, an HMO or other entity owning the hospital and employing the physicians would thereafter be treated as a single firm and would thus escape further antitrust scrutiny of its internal relationships.

A looser arrangement under which the hospital and physicians remained independent for some purposes but joined together to operate and participate in a single fully integrated enterprise might avoid antitrust interference in the operation of the joint venture itself, but the parties would have to accept continuing antitrust attention to their relationships with each other and with the joint venture entity. Even though such a joint undertaking may have been lawful at the outset, the agreement to operate it is ongoing and could be declared illegal at a later date if its implications for competition, including the venture's ability to survive without the support of its parents, should change. Finally, as long as the physicians participating in a joint venture maintain their independence for some purposes, the joint venture remains subject to antitrust oversight to ensure that it does not suppress competition beyond the point justified by the procompetitive purposes of the venture. Thus, as long as integration is not complete, some antitrust scrutiny of arrangements among the various parties necessarily continues. One hopes, however, that the courts will not go beyond requiring reasonable protection against anticompetitive abuse and will avoid demanding the adoption of a "less restrictive alternative" whenever a court can imagine one.

In *Arizona v. Maricopa County Medical Society*, the Supreme Court refused to permit a group of physicians to claim that their price-fixing agreement was a valid ancillary restraint unless they could show that the arrangement to which it was incidental was one in which they shared risks, produced a distinctive product or service, or integrated their practices. Although this holding may dichotomize too much between joint ventures and naked restraints, the idea that the degree of integration affects the applicable antitrust test is a valid one. Unfortunately, much of the law of antitrust is premised on a belief that there are only two tests, either a per se rule or a rule of reason requiring detailed inquiry into all the circumstances. Common sense and judicial practice suggest, however, that factual differences do in fact lead, and should lead, to different levels of scrutiny. As earlier discussion indicated, the relationship that exists between a hospital and its independent medical staff, if not a conspiracy to advance physician interests, may still be close enough to obviate detailed scrutiny of the resulting business decisions. On the other hand, only a tightly integrated joint venture in which the parties surrender their autonomy can hope to escape all antitrust oversight.

The lesson for hospital-physician joint ventures would appear to be that the parties must be prepared to submit fully to the control of their common enterprise if they wish to enjoy the freedom enjoyed by a single firm to carry on its business without being treated as an ongoing combination of competitors whose day-to-day actions are subject to examination as possible restraints of trade. Because autonomy is so highly prized by health care providers, designing arrangements that are safe from antitrust scrutiny may prove to be very difficult indeed.

Response

PAUL ROGERS

As we move into new organizations and as new organizations are formed by the situation we find ourselves in now, all of the points that were mentioned in Professor Havighurst's paper should be carefully analyzed. You will have to be careful of antitrust laws, although under the Reagan administration they're not too often enforced.

There has been some agreement in our discussions that the DRG law may, in effect, bring the doctor and the administrator together as they've never been brought together before. Maybe we ought to be optimistic rather than pessimistic.

Many of the major institutions of our country are going to have to go out and establish satellites and outreach facilities to feed in a patient load and to lay the foundation for the future. Bob Butler, when he was director of the National Institution of Aging, estimated that by the year 2020 or 2030, 75 percent of a doctor's time will be spent administering to those aged sixty and above.

We're already beginning to see increasing use of home health care. So tertiary care institutions are going to have to put out the satellites and they're going to have to move into home health care. Maybe this excess of doctors will be a blessing. It's coming just when we're having to do something about costs. Maybe we ought to be optimistic about that. Professor Havighurst was. Did you notice that in his comment he said a second factor affecting hospital-physician relationships is the recent growth in physician supply: "Hospitals have always needed doctors. For the first time, however, they are now able to acquire them in something other than a seller's market with the result that a doctor's willingness to cooperate in helping the hospital solve its cost problem is becoming a factor in the award of admitting privileges."

Response

MICHAEL BROMBERG

Professor Havighurst made the point that hospitals are a business and he thinks the law should look on them as a business, not as a public utility. I think that's an important point for several reasons, and from it stem several side issues.

First, the old rules of financing health care fostered looking at hospitals and their medical staffs as separate entities. In fact, hospital managers were there to please physicians. The cost reimbursement system fostered and encouraged that.

Suddenly, we're faced with new rules based on fixed revenues and fixed resources. This situation is designed to persuade hospital managers to persuade physicians to change their behavior. So far, the rules have changed with regard to the hospitals, but the old rules still apply to physicians in terms of how they generate costs in the hospital setting. If hospitals are to look at themselves as a business, their incentive will be to get physicians in the same position they're in. They won't accomplish this through changes in the law, but by joining together as partners in a risk situation. Risk is the key variable now, and risk can come in many ways—not just the traditional HMO risk, but many joint ventures that we haven't even thought about.

Second, the minute you look at any system such as hospitals as a business, antitrust laws are going to be applied to them the same way they are applied to all other businesses.

Third, whenever you have a situation in which there is a new regulatory system—and application of the antitrust law is a form of regulation of the economy—there are going to be those who seek exemptions from it. Over the last three years, the commercial insurance industry has made a visible effort to become exempt from the antitrust laws for purposes of data collection. The reason they wanted to become exempt was so that they could band together to set rates for hospitals, something we view as fairly dangerous. But it won't be just the insurance industry that looks at exemptions. It will also be those hospitals that don't like the competitive environment.

We are in a situation almost like the debate a group like this might have had two years ago, competition versus regulation. Those who don't like competition are going to want to become exempt from the antitrust laws, just as they want to be treated as a public utility rather than as a business.

Fourth, perhaps the most interesting question of all on privileges for physicians will be whether, under these new sets of incentives, hospitals will have to continue to go through the pretense of denying privileges on the grounds of quality or whether they will be able to just come right out and say, "We're a business, and for economic reasons solely, because this physician is a high utilizer and he's going to hurt us economically, we deny him privileges."

The fifth point is that the horizontal and vertical integration is going to cause the Federal Trade Commission and the Justice Department and others to look much more closely at hospitals—not just for-profit hospitals but nonprofit hospital systems as well, and their growth locally, regionally, nationally, and otherwise.

The hospital industry just sat by on the sidelines while issues of this nature arose in Congress, but the medical profession was very much involved. I think hospitals have to become more involved in the future. The Federal Trade Commission has a great deal of jurisdiction over for-profit entities. Nonprofit hospitals might be exempt from the Federal Trade Commission jurisdiction, but they are not exempt from Justice Department jurisdiction. That is something we all ought to keep in mind.

There are other legal obstacles to the formation of competitive organizations and, if hospitals have the kinds of incentives to get physicians to join with them in joint ventures and other forms of competitive alternatives, those other obstacles are going to have to be looked at closely. The state of California abolished some of those freedom of choice, insurance law, and antitrust obstacles to allow the formation of preferred provider organizations. I think that possibility is going to be looked at increasingly in other states and federally.

Based on everything I've heard so far, it sounds as if hospitals are being given every incentive to enter into the insurance market. If our incentive is to gain the cooperation of physicians in a joint venture in order to share risks, what we're really looking at is an insurance system. If that is the case, we really ought to concentrate a little more on the change to shared risk rather than what structure it takes.

Lastly, I think Mr. Rogers is correct in saying that in this Reagan administration and maybe future ones we won't see antitrust laws enforced federally. But I think we will see an incredible acceleration of antitrust application to health care at the state level and in private treble damage suits.

Discussion

DR. AFFELDT: Professor Havighurst gave a very thoughtful and scholarly analysis and presentation, but it is my interpretation that his article tells how to use the courts to restructure the relationship between hospitals and physicians to shift the power of physicians to the hospitals. But in so doing, he sees a barrier, namely JCAH. He states that the JCAH mandates an independent, self-governing medical staff. Self-governing, yes. Independent, no. I believe he has made a significant error in his analysis on that point.

Nowhere in the standards of JCAH do we refer to an independent medical staff, and yet Professor Havighurst repeatedly refers to an independent medical staff. On the contrary, our standards clearly delineate the accountability of the medical staff to the governing body.

Professor Havighurst states:

> It appears that hospitals' internal structures have been prescribed by the JCAH, a body dominated by representatives of powerful medical organizations. . . . The almost universal neglect of such alternatives for lawfully and efficiently organizing a hospital without an independent medical staff strongly suggests that the medical profession, working largely through the JCAH in recent years, has effectively controlled the terms upon which hospitals may deal with physicians.

JCAH accredits hundreds of hospitals that do not follow the model that he alludes to, including several you heard about earlier—the Henry Ford Hospital, VA hospitals, military hospitals, and public hospitals.

To further reinforce the feeling that Professor Havighurst has zeroed in on JCAH as a target, I quote from a speech he gave on

January 28, 1984, at a Conference on Hospital-Medical Public Policy Issues sponsored by the American Association of Hospital Planning: "Hospitals need freedom to develop new and innovative organizational structures to control costs. It's about time hospitals told JCAH to go to hell!"

Later at that same session, someone asked him about his comment and why he felt that way about JCAH and he responded: "I didn't like the JCAH because it could set any standard it wanted without judicial scrutiny, that JCAH's real problem was its basic sponsorship."

Our standards at JCAH have been reviewed by the Justice Department and the FTC and, most recently, the FTC requested from us and we provided the drafts of the medical staff standards from our files.

DR. SAMMONS: While we're correcting the record, Professor Havighurst talks about the five doctors in a Texas town who were recently successfully sued by the FTC for attempting to dictate a hospital's decisions. That is a misinterpretation of the facts and the circumstances.

JCAH is not guilty of all of the things that are implied here. Without a JCAH there is no voluntary accreditation agency in this country to look at and attempt to provide a vehicle for the careful evaluation and accreditation of hospitals.

I come to many of the same conclusions that Professor Havighurst made about the need for changes in the laws and in the application of some of the laws presently on the books. But I disagree with him about the due process. It may be that doctors do not have any greater right to due process than anyone else does under the law. But considering the severity of the actions taken and their implications as they apply to human life and patient care, I would have to urge that all of the efforts for due process be enhanced and reinforced in dealings between doctors and their employers.

Out of all of Professor Havighurst's study of the antitrust laws, one important point that he does make—one that we have pursued so diligently—is the redefinition of the rule of reason and the ability to apply the rule of reason. I certainly hope that he and all of the lawyers in the country who share his views will unite to do that. There is a tremendous need for a reinterpretation and redefinition and reapplication of the rule of reason in antitrust suits. However one goes about getting that done, we will all be infinitely better off when that has happened.

PROFESSOR HAVIGHURST: As far as telling the JCAH to go to hell, I had a sleepy audience of hospital administrators. In order to underscore what I was trying to say, I did use the expression. My point was that hospitals ought to consider ignoring the JCAH and arranging their internal affairs without getting the permission of the commission. On the other hand, I strongly defend the right of organizations that are involved in credentialing and accrediting to have any standard that they want. I also defend the standard that was recently repealed that would have denied accreditation to hospitals that allowed nonphysicians to admit patients. I believe an accrediting body, like the JCAH, is within its rights to maintain such a rule and the courts had no business in second-guessing such rules.

I will go back to my paper and review the use of the word "independent." I didn't really mean it as anything except a synonym for self-governing, but perhaps there is a distinction. In the future I shall be a little more alert to it.

On the rule of reason, I think we would probably agree on the change that you would like to see in the rule of reason. I think that the rule of reason ought to be rather rigorously enforced on the basis of whether it is applied and its effect on competition, not on whether there was some wording purpose being served by a particular strength, which is where the problem is.

On the subject of the physician who is left out in the cold, my sense is that if we're going to demand that hospitals be efficiently run, they must also be spared the high cost of getting rid of a physician or other provider. That is, they must be spared the risk of litigation and the necessity of bearing the burden of proving that that provider is somehow a "bad apple."

6

A New Partnership: Physicians, Hospitals, and Their Customers

DONALD S. MACNAUGHTON

"Physicians and Hospitals: The Great Partnership at a Cross-roads" is indeed a timely topic. More so than at any other time since 1966, we are seeing changes, experimentation, and the potential for significant, positive industry reform. The stage is set for hospitals and physicians to operate with new fiscal rules that create incentives for more cost efficient operations. As providers reorient their thinking and behavior, new alliances are being formed. Simply put, we are witnessing the early stages of a transformation where health services organizations are becoming more market oriented and cost effective.

Initiatives for hospitals and physicians to operate more cost efficiently are not new to the public policy agenda. A long string of legislative and regulatory initiatives have been implemented over the past decade. I refer to Medicare reimbursement limits—the so-called "223 limits"—certificate of need, PSROs, and HMO legislation. These government initiatives were, in large part, based upon good intentions—a genuine interest in solving the health care cost problem. However, these programs have fallen short of the mark. The Medicare 223 limits have shifted costs to private payers; CON has created a rather expensive market for hospital franchises and by most accounts has failed to affect hospital capital expenditures; PSROs have, with few exceptions, failed to influence medical practice; and HMO legislation of 1974 has been replaced with efforts to stimulate private investment in HMOs.

I believe that the intended purposes of these initiatives will be

This paper was presented by Mr. David G. Williamson, Executive Vice President of Development, Hospital Corporation of America.

achieved as a result of market pressures for a more cost effective health care system. Moreover, these market pressures are the driving forces behind the changes in relationships which we are here to discuss.

In the long run, society's interests will always prevail. Society demands access to quality health care at affordable prices. Attempts to achieve this objective through government fiat have not succeeded, and a strategy embracing market forces has been adopted.

I. The New Partnership

As we explore "the great partnership at the crossroads" we need to recognize that the old partnership now includes a new partner—the group purchasers of health services. This involves such diverse entities as health benefits managers of self-insured corporations, the medical czar, and business coalitions, as well as the traditional group purchasers.

The emergence of group purchasers of health services as active, more informed, and more sophisticated buyers of medical and hospital services produces three notable results. First, it puts the economic equation of buyers and sellers more in balance.

Second, purchasers assume more control through direct negotiations with providers. In the process, purchasers give basic market signals to providers, impose economic constraints on the previously unbounded definition of medical necessity, and steer employees and dependents to those providers who, in their opinion, operate more efficiently.

Third, active purchasers create an environment within which physicians' and hospitals' financial destinies are more closely linked than in the past. Previously, hospitals and physicians benefited by providing more services even though they tended to operate independently of one another. The new partnership provides both hospitals and physicians with incentives to work as partners in delivering more cost effective services to patients represented by group purchasers. Failure to meet purchasers' expectations will, in marketplaces with options, lead to lost patient volumes.

The relationship between hospitals and physicians is pressured in many ways. The initial point and controlling issue that I am attempting to present is that the most significant development in the new partnership is the changing role of the group purchaser, who is no longer a "silent" partner. Hospitals and physicians will be challenged to work constructively with their new partner, to be more market oriented. Few businesses succeed by ignoring or antagonizing their customers, and health care providers are not exceptions to this rule.

II. Cost, Quality, and Hospital Solvency

Before overviewing three relationships, let me address the under-lying trade-offs between cost, quality, and hospital solvency. As hospital managers and physicians respond to cost pressures, hospital structures and behavior will change. There is no layer of fat to absorb significant cost cuts without notice. Something will be sacrificed. Let me now address three factors relating to hospital costs.

First the quality issue. In Economics 101 we learned that cost equals price times quantity and, further, when price is controlled and quantity ignored, we have a problem. In health care, this translates to the diminution of quality. Consequently the crucible for the new partnership relates to its ability to assure continuity of quality through the judicious and appropriate utilization of re-sources. This could be the factor that places the greatest strain on partner relationships.

The second factor related to cost is that of cross-subsidization. While most industries support some level of cross-subsidization, the hospital industry supports major social policies by shifting costs. Graduate medical education, services provided to indigent patients, Medicare and Medicaid beneficiaries, and low volume services (e.g., obstetrical, emergency room, etc.) contribute to the amount of cross-subsidization in hospital charge structures. Cost pressures induced by competition or rate regulation reduce a hos-pital's ability to continue this practice. To the extent that these social policies remain important, explicit financing will be re-quired.

The last factor is the set of amenities involved in health ser-vices delivery. During the cost-based reimbursement era of the past seventeen years, amenity levels of many hospitals have im-proved. Modern plants and equipment, private rooms, more con-venient locations, patient communication systems, carpeting, high levels of nurse staffing, etc., are more commonplace in hos-pitals. Generally speaking, amenities are currently equally acces-sible by all patients. However, we are seeing more attention to different categories of patients defined by the level of payment.

Cost pressures will be felt unevenly across different patient groups, creating incentives to vary amenity levels. This gets at the subject of a multitiered system, in which there is agreement that clinical quality should not be compromised. However, differences in amenity levels provided to varying groups of patients will undoubtedly become more visible as hospitals respond to cost pressures.

It is unclear how hospitals and physicians will ultimately deal with these factors in response to cost pressures, but something will be lost when costs are reduced. It is reasonable to suspect that all hospitals will strive to remain fiscally viable, but that in an industry that has excess capacity, some hospitals will not survive.

In the airline industry we recently witnessed the combination of cost pressures (induced by price competition) and excess capacity leading to reduced capacity. Some firms reduced capacity in a managed fashion; however, significant industry wide adjustments occurred when a few major carriers went bankrupt.

The hospital industry will likely face some of the same challenges as airline companies. Two important questions are raised by these prospects. First, to what extent will the "market test" be allowed to determine which hospitals survive? When Braniff filed for bankruptcy, we did not see the outcry that is likely to occur if a major community hospital files for bankruptcy. Second, how will the public be safeguarded when a hospital has exhausted its cost-cutting options in the amenities and cross-subsidization categories? At what point do the traditional professional safeguards of licensure, accreditation, and peer review need strengthening because of the financial condition of providers?

At this juncture, it would be exceedingly difficult to lay out a general prescription for reducing health care costs while maintaining quality and ensuring hospital solvency. The complexity of the trade-offs should be apparent, as should the need to move cautiously in our quest for a more cost effective health delivery system.

III. Three Key Relationships

Changes in the medical marketplace are redefining relationships between the major actors. I will focus on three of these relationships: the hospital-physician relationship; the group purchasers-provider relationship; and the hospital-hospital relationship.

A. HOSPITAL-PHYSICIAN

The hospital-physician relationship is a cornerstone of the health care delivery system. The traditionally cooperative relationship is now being tested, as physicians and hospitals see their individual interests increasingly diverge from their mutual interests. Opportunities are emerging for both to proceed as allies or competitors.

The emerging hospital-physician relationship is not likely to be uniform across the country. The resulting relationships will be influenced by several factors.

1. Geography. The rural areas with single hospitals and an appropriate physician supply will witness less strain on relationships than metropolitan areas with multiple facilities and excesses in physician manpower. Moreover, the rural areas are less likely to witness the quantity of alternative delivery systems or financing options such as HMOS, PPOS, and the like.

2. Quality of historical relationships. Hospitals that have a history of fragile relationships with physicians are not apt to enjoy a good one in an increasingly competitive environment.

3. The large multihospital organizations. These organizations, which have access to capital and the ability to market both institutional and physician services on a national scale, will have better opportunities to maintain a symbiotic relationship with physicians.

The changing competitive environment will not only produce winners and losers in an economic sense, but winners and losers with respect to hospital-physician relationships. The following suggest some characteristics of the winners: the ones that define and mutually agree upon the appropriate role for each to play; the ones that innovate and discover new methods to respond to the message of the marketplace; the ones that understand that the individual physician's goal and agenda are not always consistent with those of the institution and that some conflict and adverse behavior can redound to the benefit of patients and society in general; and the ones that acknowledge that long-term relationships can best be built through philosophical and programmatic joint efforts as opposed to economic joint ventures.

B. GROUP PURCHASERS-PROVIDERS

As insurance companies, health benefit managers, and the administrators of the Medicare and Medicaid programs complete their evolution from fiscal conduits to more active purchasers of health services, their relationship with hospitals and physicians will change as well. Currently, both providers and purchasers are in the early stages of their new roles. Employers and insurance companies, frustrated by rising health care costs, are experimenting with approaches to cost containment. This experimentation includes expanding their relationship with providers. At the same time, hospitals and physicians are in the midst of adjusting to new financial ground rules. Combined, the situations are best described as confusing. Let me first focus on some new considerations each faces with respect to the relationships.

Employers are coming to grips with their responsibility for managing health benefit expenditures. Organized efforts through the Business Roundtable, the National Chamber of Commerce, the Washington Business Group on Health, local business health coalitions, and individual companies all suggest a multitude of initiatives. These range from understanding services options to benefit restructuring, health promotion programs, and selection of preferred provider groups. While many companies have already undertaken such initiatives, it is accurate to characterize their situation as "still being at the high end of the learning curve." They are in the process of learning the basics of dealing with health care providers either directly or through insurance companies; still learning how to articulate what products they really want; and honing their negotiating skills. Utilization review programs, outpatient surgery, steering of patients, pricing, guaranteed volumes, quick payment cycles, etc., are emerging as the focal points of these discussions. Many of these initiatives establish a "gatekeeper" function that is separate from the traditional role of the private physician. Health care providers are learning how to shift from a "more is better" to a "more efficient is better" orientation. They are grappling with new organization vehicles for working together, marketing themselves to purchasers, and developing the managerial tools necessary to operate in the new environment.

There are as yet no clear indications of a single type of relationship developing between purchasers and providers. It is encouraging that a constructive dialogue is occurring on many fronts. Lessons from other buyer-seller relationships suggest that the best results tend to emerge when both parties approach negotiations expecting mutual benefits and work toward long run relationships focusing on quality, value, and price. Attempts to stimulate destructive price wars, attempts to drive suppliers out of business, and barriers to open communication tend to work against both parties.

The many purchasers assuming responsibility for managing health benefit expenditures also assume the role of a control mechanism that I believe collectively will precipitate significant positive industry reforms. Unfortunately, there are companies and associations avoiding this responsibility by seeking such government intervention as rate setting and "all payers systems" as the solution to the health care cost problem. I believe such government actions would be misguided and counterproductive to the development of a cost effective health care system. I further suspect that, in those states with heavy-handed regulatory programs, group purchasers have less freedom and less ability to work and negotiate with providers to their own advantage.

We face a number of important public policy issues related to further evolution of the active group purchaser. These include the impact of government regulation on developments in the medical marketplace, the emergence of a more blatant multitiered health care system, the willingness of private purchasers to continue subsidizing public goods through cost shifting, and the willingness of government to explicitly finance social policies they have legislated.

C. HOSPITAL-HOSPITAL RELATIONSHIPS

There are a number of new and innovative relationships emerging between hospitals that are significant in and of themselves but that also have implications for physician relationships.

Lessons from other industries that recently became more price competitive (e.g., financial services, trucking, real estate, etc.) suggest that successful companies tend to adopt one or more of three distinct strategies. They form or join national full service companies with broad marketing and distribution capabilities; they specialize in definable niches; and/or they compete in some niche at the low cost end of the market.

We are already seeing similar developments in the health care industry. First, multiple hospital systems, both national and regional, both investor-owned and not-for-profit, continue to develop geographical networks. Freestanding hospitals are undergoing corporate restructuring to integrate vertically within a defined marketplace. Hospital Corporation of America represents not only a multi-hospital system, but one that is entering into joint venture arrangements with major teaching institutions and formally tying itself to medical research through venture capital programs and select vendor projects.

The specialization strategy is occurring in the sense that private psychiatric hospitals, women's hospitals, orthopedic hospitals, rehabilitation hospitals, oncology hospitals, etc., are becoming more prominent. In addition, hospitals under DRGs are shedding services thus leaving a smaller number of major specialty areas as the hospital's "product."

The low cost providers are currently less pronounced. Nevertheless, chains of outpatient activities including surgicenters, imaging centers, regional labs, etc., represent one form of this development. And some hospital systems have declared themselves to be operating in the low-cost, highly efficient end of the hospital marketplace.

It is not clear how far such segmentation will go in the health care industry, but the trend toward consolidation and networking of facilities seems to cut across all three strategies. This offers the promise of better access to capital, economies of scale, and the opportunity to market more effectively to group purchasers.

This networking of hospitals will also create pressures to change traditional physician referral patterns and staff privileges. There are no general conclusions to be reached about these issues, but they again emphasize the importance of physicians and hospitals working as allies and partners.

As we make the transition to a more cost effective system, we will continue to face many challenges. Redefining relationships that have been reinforced over decades is no simple task. We must strive to remain professional and cooperative. Health care after all is a service with important social, political, legal, and economic overtones. Our approach to the changes we face must be cautious and balanced. If we succeed, we will end this decade having regained public confidence and possessed of a health care delivery system of which we can all be proud.

Response

UWE E. REINHARDT

Mr. MacNaughton argues that the driving force behind the impending changes is the group purchaser of health services: the health benefit managers, medical czars, insurance companies, and so on. He feels that the force of these purchasers will drive doctors and hospitals closer together. That, of course, is a hypothesis. I'm not sure whether it will drive them closer together or split them apart.

He mentions that there is no fat to absorb significant cuts in costs, so that something will have to give, something will have to be sacrificed, perhaps quality. A question that comes to mind is, exactly what does he mean by quality? It's not clear to me exactly how the term quality is interpreted in his discussion. Are we talking about the clinical quality of the service or the social quality of the system? Those are two different things.

Imagine clinical quality on a vertical axis, that is, the medical quality of services delivered to those who actually get them. Then, on the horizontal axis, imagine social quality, that is, the percent of people actually reached by the health service sector with a given clinical quality. You can opt for a system that has very high clinical quality but doesn't reach all the people or for a system that sacrifices some clinical quality but reaches more people. The American health sector has generally emphasized the clinical quality while somewhat deemphasizing the social quality of health care, while the British system seems to sacrifice some clinical quality for the sake of social quality. So, when we talk about the market driven system, what exactly is it that we're talking about?

I don't really care very much what kind and on what terms rich people like us get health care. The real problem that makes health care a public policy issue has always been the social problem of welding the market ethic to a quite different social ethic.

We have here a business—a hospital—that is a multiproduct firm with high fixed costs and low variable costs. Every time you have high fixed costs and low direct variable costs you have a situation ripe for price discrimination, which the insurance industry calls cost shifting. When you fly TWA from New York to the west coast, you have rampant cost shifting of the overhead: not one person in the plane is likely to pay the same fare as another.

When group purchasers exert their muscle to bargain for good deals, that means that some big, powerful groups get better prices than less powerful groups. Twenty million Americans are now uninsured: they're the ones with the least market power and presumably they will bear the overhead.

People complain about cost shifting. Cost shifting in American health care has been the saving grace of that system in order to camouflage an American disgrace—that is, twenty million uninsured Americans.

Mr. McNaughton mentions that the amenities will vary in hospitals by ability to pay, but that the clinical quality will not. How can he be sure that is so? Or, if he can be sure it is so, how can he be sure that the people won't correlate low amenities with poor medical quality? What will be the social response to this? With TWA, we have first, ambassador, and coach classes, and people put up with that, but will they in a hospital? Or will that not trigger one of the waves in this cybernetic feedback that Dr. Wallace spoke about? One of the waves might bring on a quite strong reaction.

When you talk about cost effectiveness and efficiency, you must realize that just reducing cost doesn't tell you anything about efficiency at all. You may have simply redistributed quality.

In these proceedings we have treated the hospital as a business. I recently did a survey on how other nations finance hospital capital, and the one thing that stunned me is that there isn't another nation on earth that thinks about a hospital as a business the way we do. There isn't a nation on earth that doesn't view the hospital as a community service, a quasi-extension of the government or the community, and therefore feel entitled to plan that sector and obligated to finance it. We view it as a business.

You've got to keep in mind what a business corporation is. The other day, in my freshman class, I asked, "What is the social responsibility of a business corporation?" and I said, "I can put it very simply in one sentence. It's to maximize shareholders' wealth without violating the laws of the land!" There is no other social responsibility.

There are indications here for a for-profit sector. You have to understand the social limits of for-profit medicine. It cannot do certain things that need to be done.

And then you have to ask yourself, "How do we then deal with the economic misfits?" Those are the people who cannot fend for themselves in the market because their intellect isn't sharp enough, or they're sick, or they were born into poverty. The only option we really have is to deliver health care to them through the privately owned corporations, but then pricing rears its ugly head. How do you then buy from the private sector the services for the economic misfits? If you don't, you'll have to have public delivery with public financing and you will have two parallel hospital systems: one for public patients and one private.

I recently read in a Morgan Stanley report of one hospital: "Improvements will be achieved by staffing cutbacks, reducing the average length of stay, attracting a more profitable patient mix. Corporate overhead should be reduced."

That kind of language is uniquely American, and it may be for the good. I'm not sure the American people will stand for it, though, unless you worry about the twenty million or so people who cannot fend for themselves in that sort of system. If I were the for-profit hospital sector, that's the one problem I would really worry about, because that's where the explosion is likely to come if one ever does come.

Response

ALAIN ENTHOVEN

First, to comment on the changing character on the demand side, Mr. MacNaughton wrote that market pressures are demanding a more cost-effective health care system; that group purchasers of health care are emerging as a new partner, more active, more informed, and more sophisticated than before, even though still on the high and steep end of the learning curves, even though many of them are just beginning to look at health care.

In the past, organized medicine succeeded in enforcing the principles of fee-for-service, cost reimbursement and so-called free choice of doctor, and that equates to cost-unconscious demand. That is, insurers were not able to negotiate selectively for price, utilization, and quality, because by law they couldn't control the patient's choice of provider and, therefore, they had no bargaining power.

When these principles were combined with society's desire for comprehensive health insurance—expressed as a tax subsidy through provided health insurance, Medicare and Medicaid—a condition was created in the marketplace that Martin Feldstein once characterized as "permanent excess demand." In that environment, buyers had little hope of being able to control the clinical quality or the cost of care. Now that is breaking down. The costs got too high. The government could not afford cost-unconscious demand for its beneficiaries. As the government changed its behavior with respect to the purchasers for its own beneficiaries, employers, fearing a massive cost shift, have also started to make more selective provider-contracting for their own beneficiaries. They have brought pressure on legislators to break down some of the restrictive legislation that made it impossible for them to insert cost-conscious demands before. In California in 1982, for example, we passed a law that repealed a prohibition on insurance companies negotiating selectively for rates and utilization and directing patients to preferred providers.

One important characteristic about the new demand side will be purchaser interest in more global units of care. I think that that is a step toward economic efficiency; that is, payers will want to start to buy in units whose price and clinical quality they can understand and compare. Providers, on the other hand, if they're selling broader, more global units of care, have the opportunity to allocate resources to produce those more global units of care in the most efficient way.

Prices for services as we're seeing in preferred provider organizations and the prospective payment system of diagnosis related groups fall short of the ideal of economic efficiency in the sense of making a contract that allows the least costly way of achieving the desired product. In the long run, I think the adjusted cost per capita will prove to be a far more satisfactory denominator on the basis of which buyers will want to buy care. Cost per capita rewards providers for keeping people out of the hospital and away from high cost DRGs. Cost per capita systematically involves physicians in total costs. It makes payment independent of the process of care because you don't have problems like coding DRG treatment and the like. It is simpler and easier to understand and it implies a contractual obligation to care for members of an enrolled population.

One of the serious problems with prospective payment by DRG, with very wide variations in the cost per case within a given DRG, is that there will be very serious pressure for hospitals to dump the severe cases. They won't be inhibited from doing so, because there will be no contractual obligation on the part of the providers to take care of that patient. One thing I find comforting in being a member of an HMO is that no matter how bad I look, those providers have a contractual obligation to take care of me.

Another important characteristic on the demand side in this new market is that it will be more conscious of clinical quality measure by outcomes. As employers move to limit choice of employees, they will find that they are going to be held responsible for the quality of the selected providers. In the past, employers have had nothing to do with quality because they've had nothing to do with selecting the provider. They've given their employees a financial hunting license for a doctor. Now when they start limiting their employees' choices they're responsible for picking good doctors and excluding bad ones. Employers are going to need to be credible on the question of quality in order to induce employees to willingly accept a limited choice and to see it in positive terms and not as a negative restraint.

Clinical quality of care is in the employer's interest. It means less sick leave, less disability, early return of healthy workers, satisfied employees, and the like. Selective contracting will give the employer tools to control quality that haven't been available in the past. As a result, the concept of quality will be more statistical and more population-based and less based on pedigree and credentials. Employers will think of quality the way they do in their own businesses, statistically measuring what comes off the production line and seeing how many mistakes there are. Cutting costs in such a milieu will not usually mean cutting the quality of care. On the contrary, quality and economy will go more hand in hand. After all, the best care is the most economical care in the long run.

John Young of Hewlett-Packard wrote an article a few years ago about how Hewlett-Packard went about cutting costs and he said, "What we discovered as the most economical thing to do is to do it right the first time!" I think that will become more and more evident in medical care. The right diagnosis done promptly, the procedure done correctly by a proficient provider with low rates of complications. Quality is expensive and the providers will try harder when they have to pay for their own mistakes, which is something that will happen under this new kind of demand. More and more providers will be under prepaid capital financing where their own mistakes in the form of complications and the like fall back on them instead of leading to higher fees and charges.

I disagree with Mr. MacNaughton's implication that if you cut spending you're somehow going to sacrifice something. I believe it will be possible to cut costs substantially by improving the cost of care and eliminating waste, and the way to do this will be through systematic data gathering and evaluation.

What has all this to say about the theme of our conference with respect to relationships between hospitals and doctors? What I'm offering is a sort of economic and managerial view of that relationship.

I think these market forces, these changing characters on the demand side will mean greater integration of physicians and hospitals in order to maximize efficiency. As Mr. MacNaughton said, this active purchaser creates an environment within which physicians' and hospitals' financial destinies are more closely linked than in the past. I think they'll become tightly linked through the competitive medical plans in which they will participate and, increasingly, effective integration will be needed to maximize efficiency. For example, quality assurance will mean measuring outcomes over a long term. Pressures for quality assurance will mean measuring outcomes over a long-term follow-up and asking patients how they perceive the results of their care in order to evaluate the costs, risks, and benefits of treatments. That will require shared unit medical records maintained over a substantial period of time.

Improved efficiency means matching the resources used to the needs of the population served, both in the aggregate and by time of day. That means control of the numbers of doctors and specialties to assure busy schedules and to assure proficiency. If you have too many neurosurgeons in town, at best that means a lot of nonproficient neurosurgeons and, at worst, it might mean a combination of that and too much neurosurgery. Efficient scheduling of doctors means efficient scheduling of their whole time to meet patient demand. That will take full-time players on the cost effective team, at least if they intend to be winners in this competition. This is also going to mean a systematic peer review of outcomes and of resource use, and corrective action will be taken with respect to the poor performers.

Another reason for greater integration is the fact that you cannot have cost-unconscious culture heroes in a cost-effective organization. What the efficient organization that meets this new market is going to need is a shared culture that includes quality assurance and cost effectiveness. Doctors, hospitals and competitive medical plans will have to develop a winning quality and cost-conscious culture and that means more integration. They will have to optimize operations for total effectiveness so that, for instance, the lab tests come back at a time that's consistent with a short stay in the hospital. The setting in which care is delivered will have to yield to cost-effective choice: surgicenters, home care, and so forth. The financial incentives will have to be brought into congruence with organizational goals. You cannot have a cost-effective organization if you reward behavior that is opposed to the organizational goal of better quality care at lower cost. We cannot have a straight, unattenuated, fee-for-procedure system with no incentive for economy.

Physicians will, of course, remain the key players on the team. You simply cannot have a good medical care program without them. But competitive pressures for efficiency will necessitate closer teamwork between physicians and hospitals.

Finally, I would like to comment on Professor Reinhardt's thought provoking remarks on the question of how we deal with economic misfits and can we reconcile equity in the search for efficiency that is produced by a competitive marketplace. I think that the subsidies that ought to be made available by society to the economic misfits ought to be explicit and they ought to be equitable. In fact, I've recently written an article proposing a restructuring of the tax subsidies. Today, the federal government is losing about $30 billion a year in revenue in tax subsidies to employer-provided health insurance. These subsidies are worth much more to the high income, well insured, well-to-do than to low-income people who don't have the benefit of powerful employee groups. One of the proposals I made, which I think would move in the direction Professor Reinhardt would like to see us go, is that we make those subsidies explicit and we make them available to low-income people as well as to high-income people. I would like to think that we would even go further and make even more subsidies available. Through explicit subsidies, we ought to assure everyone's financial access. Government purchasers should purchase for the poor and for the indigent. In our society it is a fairly ambitious task to hope that government could do that well, but I don't agree with the suggestion that you cannot have a market system and equity at the same time. I am afraid, on the contrary, that if we do not use the market to achieve some efficiency, we will never be able to afford an equitable system.

Discussion

MR. BROMBERG: Morris Abrams said recently that there is a difference between two-track and two-tier medicine. Two-tier medicine suggests that poor people are getting lower quality clinical care. Two-track medicine, which is okay at least from the ethics point of view, says that the amenities may not be equally good but the quality of the clinical care is.

Two examples of two-track medicine are public hospitals, where the quality of medical care is excellent in a teaching environment but the amenities may not be as good, and the neighborhood health clinic, where poor people have access to health care. My point is that you do not have to sacrifice access. Perhaps the most interesting point in Mr. MacNaughton's paper is his suggestion that in order to preserve access we may have to think in terms of different levels of amenities. This is not two-tier or multitier medicine; it's multitrack medicine.

The second point I wanted to address was the concern that, if the group purchaser becomes the new player in this partnership and starts to demand discounts, that will do terrible things to the limited group including the twenty million uninsured. Instead of thinking about shifting costs to make up for the discount, maybe we need to look at ways to cut costs.

The one point I would disagree with in Mr. MacNaughton's paper is his contention that there is no fat to cut from hospital costs. There is, and to the extent that there is, we can hold down the growth of employees and make sure wage and benefit increases aren't higher than in other fields. Those actions are not just going to benefit Medicare or Ford Motor Company. They are going to benefit everybody, because costs are costs to everyone.

The same thing for medical utilization. We are not just going to see reduced length of stay for one payer. If it works, it is going to work across the board.

I think we can give discounts without hurting the twenty million poor people.

PROFESSOR REINHARDT: I don't deny that cost shifting might have some effect on costs overall, but the price differentials will remain.

Once you cut it to the bare bone, you still have high overhead and the question in economic theory then becomes, how do you optimally allocate this overhead to different classes? Who are the people who are price insensitive? They may be either people who are so rich it doesn't matter or people who are so sick they can't help it. And that is another problem.

So far we have used a device shifting cost to people who could probably bear it.

There are many possible multitier or multitrack systems to use. I usually say one is brutal, and that is what we are using now. If someone can't pay, we pretend we have a one-track or one-tier system and we balance the budget by kicking him or her out altogether. A more humane approach is a multitrack system. Multitier implies high versus low. Multitrack may be choice-constrained versus nonconstrained. It is conceivable that the choice-constrained systems are in fact better in terms of quality of care.

PROFESSOR ENTHOVEN: I just wanted to pick up on a couple of things that Mr. Bromberg said. I don't think the big dollars in health care are in the amenities. They are not in single or double or triple rooms. The big dollars are in high tech care, and I would hope that that would be equally available to the rich and the poor. I don't think we need to go to a two-tier society. We can have HMOs that cater to the "carriage trade" where you have a lovely doctor waiting at the door for you, and others where you have to wait two hours for an appointment.

The other thing is we could have something like Robinson-Patman pricing rules called community ratings so that you wouldn't have this kind of selective discount system. One of the better hospitals in our area, El Camino Hospital, refused to participate in Blue Cross, group buyer, and other similar things, saying to their purchasers that such participation was bound to cause cost shifting. If they gave a discount to Blue Cross that meant they would have to charge more to somebody else. Instead they just contract with the leading companies for one uniform efficient price. That's the way to argue from the point of view of economic efficiency.

DR. WILBUR: The question arises whether it is socially desirable in this country to allow different levels of amenities. And the answer is yes, because the clinical quality is the same.

I would disagree with Professor Enthoven who just said that amenities weren't the cause of the high cost of health care, but the high technology is. I don't think that is supportable in most economic analyses.

I would ask Mr. Williamson to tell us why Mr. MacNaughton thinks that economic joint relationships between medical staffs and the hospitals are wrong. I don't understand that. Several presentations at this conference have spoken in favor of the subject.

PROFESSOR THOMPSON: I would like to make two points. First, I would ask why in the Economics 101 section of his paper Mr. MacNaughton ignored quantity. There are economies of scale within certain DRGs, and it would seem to me that one future strategy of many hospitals will be to increase the quantity and decrease the price of selected DRGs, which was completely ignored in the paper.

Second, I completely agree with Professor Enthoven that payment on a per capita basis is the way we are going to have to go. We consider DRG as a temporary step on the road to capitation so that we can write a good policy. Right now we don't know how much it will really cost us, so it is impossible to write a good policy. There are differences in selected DRGs between the way HMO patients and non-HMO patients are treated in the hospitals, and that is very significant in projecting what the policy would cost.

MR. MCMAHON: We're beginning to see some differences of opinion so deeply imbedded in our own political, economic, and social outlook that they won't change very much, which is one of the things that makes debate useful.

We are going to have a different level of hospital-physician relationships, depending on whether we move in the direction of marketplace incentives or whether we have a more regulated environment. The latter may be the only way to get social considerations into the equation. I think hospitals are beginning to understand the public policy issue a little more clearly than physicians; that is, that there have to be changes in the way we provide medical care because the way we have been providing it leads to excessive increases in costs, problems of government deficits, and a high cost of business production.

If hospitals and their physicians cannot adjust to the realities of the current trends, we will have to bring more marketplace incentives into the system as a means of reducing the rate of increase in costs and thus responding to that public policy that is so clearly announced. Some government action will occur. Some of my constituents very clearly prefer government interference because the warm security blanket of regulation will keep them from having to deal with that most difficult of their problems, a medical staff whose leadership doesn't understand the public policy message, who resist as the pilots resisted the rules and regulations of the mother ship.

I don't care whether we're at the crossroads or not; we are some place along an evolutionary path that means that relationships will have to be different and part of the way those relationships will change will affect the regulatory environment. The regulatory environment, if we don't do something on our own, will affect that relationship for the worse.

DR. ELLWOOD: I wonder whether the multihospital systems have an advantage in striking some sort of bargain with the doctors. None of the multihospital systems controls a major alternative delivery system at the present time. The reason that they've been timid is the fear that in attempting to strike a deal with doctors in a community, they will incur some hostility in that community, and the hostility will spread throughout their system. There is a hazard of this happening right now with Humana in Louisville. Do you think that conditions are sufficiently different that the multihospital systems can now take advantage of their management and capital and geographic spread to establish economic relationships with doctors that they have been reluctant to establish in the past?

PROFESSOR ENTHOVEN: I want to comment a little about high tech costs: I am thinking, for example, of the town in which 50 percent of hospital costs were associated with 13 percent of patients and those were very sick patients. The Rand Corporation found in their randomized trial that 1 percent of the patients in their sample accounted for 28 percent of all the costs. Other studies have come up with similar numbers. What makes those people costly is partly the high technology and partly nursing time.

Whether you have one patient or four patients in a room doesn't change the cost nearly as much as the question of the severity of illness of those patients and the number of nursing hours they require and how efficiently the hospital is run.

Personally, I don't believe in a two-track system. I think we can have efficient care available for all. A fair number of people from well-to-do families on our faculty and around where I live buy happiness and good quality care in the most cost-effective and efficient health care organizations. I don't think amenities are an issue. I think the issue is the efficiency of the health care organizations. If we could reorganize the delivery systems to be efficient, it would be a lot easier for the price of these subsidies to pave the way for bringing the low income and the aged into the quality mainstream. An efficient system could easily cut 25 percent out of the costs.

PROFESSOR REINHARDT: Americans have what I call a John Wayne complex. By that I mean we always just simply assert, "We've got the best this or that; we've got the best army in the world," and so on. I have always heard this in health care, too: "We have the best health care system in the world." I don't accept that.

I once saw a film on TV called "Your Money or Your Life," which took Kings County Hospital in New York and Downstate Hospital, a university hospital, and just filmed what went on there. It's pretty sobering to see what goes on in those hospitals. I remember a lady who had to be readmitted and they said at the admitting office, "You still owe us $60 from the last hospital bill." She opened her purse and she had $72; she gave them $60 so she could be admitted, and her husband was in another hospital and she cried right into the camera. This was real and I thought, "It's funny. You cannot make such a film in Canada!" It is not wrong to remind ourselves that there is that other dimension in which we Americans have not always done as well as a rich nation could.

Mr. McMahon says he doesn't know how to get social policy in the equation. Professor Enthoven began quite beautifully doing just that. He wrote a book about it, and one beautiful thing about that book is that concern for social equity is very much the theme that runs through it.

The trouble with the market strategy that we seem to have adopted is that we took half of it but not the other half, not the social concern. There are ways of somehow making the medical care experience for America's economic misfits humane. They don't have to be the same amenities but they do have to be humane so that not only the quality of care is good but also the social experience and the financial experience aren't a disaster. That's feasible.

Economists as a professional group have never asked the government for any help of any sort. We have never asked the government to protect our professional or economic turfs through licensing. Because we didn't invite the government into our business to protect us, the government has no business being in our business. But, you in health care did. You ran to the government as a source of power every time your turf was threatened. You refused to open this market, to let para-dental and para-medical practitioners compete openly the way any para-economist can.

The minute you invite the government into your business to do anything for you at all, it also has the right to ask what you will do with that power they gave you. You are simply dreaming when you assume that the government has no right in it. They gave you a power and they have every right to see what gets done with it and what effect it has on prices.

Open this market, throw it wide open, let pediatric nurses open up and give well-baby care, allow the patients to choose, and I think there will be no more justification for government interference in your business. But you haven't done that and therefore the government has a right to be in there.

PROFESSOR LIPSCOMB: The problem of how to get some social aspects into the equation can be solved in one way as Alain Enthoven says in his book by trying to put more competition and efficiency into the system; not putting more resources into the system, but reorganizing the way the system handles the resources that it currently has. Then you can achieve greater social quality for any given level of clinical quality.

Another way, though, to achieve greater social quality is to infuse more resources into the system from the bottom side: more expenditures for Medicaid for direct purchase; more vouchers for Medicare for the elderly; negative income tax credits. By infusing more resources there would be greater purchasing power.

Both of those proposals have some difficulty. The latter proposal involves spending much much more money, and we don't seem to have the money to spend. The former proposal involves reorganizing medicine in an area in which there continues to be a very controversial and difficult set of problems.

MR. WILLIAMSON: There is some anxiety on the part of some physicians about the multihospital systems getting into alternative delivery systems. When Humana announced they were going to have six hundred "doc-in-a-box" shops throughout the country, a lot of physicians became concerned about it. The real cost to the physicians is the lost opportunity in their main line of business. One hospital in Phoenix declined from a 6.5 percent share of the market to a 4.7 percent share when a competing "doc-in-a-box" shop went into operation. There is some concern among physicians about that.

We have some concern that Ford Motor Company or Eli Lilly can suggest to physicians how they should change their behavior a little easier than we at Hospital Corporation of America can. We have established a program that we call Prime-Ed which we piloted in Nashville. We have about 7,000 employees there, and we have said to the employees, "If you go to physicians who have privileges on the staff of the six HCA hospitals in the area, we will pay 90 percent of the bill. If you go to a brand X hospital and therefore brand X doctors, you pay 70 percent of the bill." Thus we'll be in a position to help to bring physicians more patients.

In HCA's strategy statements to all hospital administrators we take the position that we will not enter into joint economic ventures with physicians. What has been suggested to us in the past is that physicians both owning hospitals and putting patients in the hospitals was somehow a conflict of interest. Now everybody seems to say that the relationships between physicians and hospitals can be salvaged if we put the physician at risk by economically joining him with us in some kind of economic venture. His prescribing power and therefore his ability to get at the health care dollar redounds to the benefit of both physicians and hospitals. I wonder whether or not it makes for a better long-lasting relationship if we do something together programmatically rather than something that will line the pockets of the physicians and hospitals at the same time.

Professor Reinhardt commented about the business of medicine and suggested that this country is the only one that thinks in that idiom. We're probably also the only industrial society in which we have private not-for-profit hospitals. Most other societies have either government hospitals or private hospitals. Social consciousness on the part of either not-for-profit or for-profit hospitals pretty much has to be the same.

The question really is not where are we going to take care of the poor and the disadvantaged. The question is, how is society going to finance it? For too long the whole discussion has centered around ownership while the real issue is how you finance the care of the poor and indigent and not where you take care of them.

7

Summary I

ELI GINZBERG

First, the title of the conference has to do with partnerships between hospitals and physicians. From my perspective, a partnership is a very strange form of business organization in the year
1984 and it will be even stranger in the year 1994. It is not one of
the generic ways in which our economy has been developing,
from which I conclude that maybe the whole field of health care
is something special and that's why the word "partnership" is on
the table. If you were thinking about the automobile industry, the
educational industry, or any other industry, you wouldn't have the
word "partnership" around the table. You cannot do anything in
the health care field without substantial concentrated resources,
such as in a hospital, and key people who are physicians, not to
mention the support staff.

You have to remember that, because otherwise we could have
had a discussion here about corporate medicine. Why wasn't it
called corporate medicine? I think for very good reasons that there
is a tradition in America that professionals, especially physicians,
don't want to be employees.

Second, I cannot agree that health care is a business. There is
no business in the United States in which 70 percent of current
expenditures are prepaid: 40 percent by the government and another 30 percent by insurance.

Third, there are a lot of changes going on in that market out
there: there is unbundling; there are new investments for ambulatory facilities; there are hospitals trying to get satellites. These
are obviously all affected by doctors who want to maintain their
income, hospitals that want to survive, and a lot of people who
want to make some money. The only conclusion I can draw from
all that activity is that people and institutions are putting more

resources into the system in order to get niches, in order to make profits, in order to protect their income, the only possible consequence of which is that the costs will continue to go up rapidly.

Somewhere in an indefinite future, conceivably, some of the excess hospitals may close, but not very soon. And, since physicians don't have a very easy time moving laterally out of the field, they are going to stay in the field. I see continuing severe cost pressures coming from lots of people scrambling to further strengthen their position.

As far as I can read the reports, the American public is basically satisfied with the health care system and wants more health care. While they keep talking about costs, they're really not much concerned about costs yet. There are employers and legislators who are concerned about costs, but the public is not, by and large.

These institutions we call nonprofit hospitals seem to belong to whatever community they are in, so you don't take them away so easily and they don't change their natures so quickly. They came out of a combination of community and philanthropy with a little bit of government help. Some of them are 200 and 250 years old, and you don't quite so cavalierly decide that they can or cannot do this, that, or the other thing.

I have always been unimpressed with the suggestion that we make great economies by taking the educational costs out of the hospital and putting them onto a different budget line. I have watched that discussion in Washington for twenty years, and it doesn't really mean anything. Educational costs have to be paid for; by the time you shift them around, you'll get something worse.

I disagree with Professor Enthoven on only one point. He has been a great believer that our tax system in the health insurance field is wrong and I agree with him. I think it's crazy. But I wouldn't spend one minute of my time recommending its change because I know that, every time you fool around with the tax system in any big way affecting a large number of workers, it won't work and you'll come out with something that's still worse! I will consider changing the hospital tax system or the insurance system when we change the depreciation on oil wells.

I come from a city where we've always had four levels of health care. We've had good care at the top; we've had second level care which was more or less passable; and then we've had care for the poor, which was not too bad; and then we've had absolutely awful care. We have always had a great big government system in addition to a very large voluntary system. So I've never understood the notion that we have one level of care in this country. Even with all the levels that we have in New York, people do not do very well but fairly well.

I looked up what the estimates were for 1983 for the total health care of seven million New Yorkers plus the one million other people who get hospitalized in New York during the course of the year: $17 billion for total health care expenditures in New York in 1983. I would love to see how the market suddenly is going to change all that. We will have only the most minute alterations in the system in the foreseeable future.

What do I see in terms of a policy agenda? I see the states becoming major controlling agents in the health care of the United States at an accelerating clip. I see state after state, because of the Medicaid commitment on the one hand and the insurance premiums on the second hand and competitive benefit costs on the third hand and a lot of other things bothering them, becoming much more active. That is another way of saying that I believe that state regulation will be moving faster than the market to bring things under control, particularly with reference to new facilities. An extreme case was in New York recently where Memorial Hospital couldn't get a nuclear magnetic resonance imaging unit and some for-profit physician in Long Island just bought himself one. That is the kind of limited state operation that won't continue for very long.

The states have to move because no politician who's elected to a state legislature can be party to uncovering the poor by closing a hospital that serves them. The political cost of doing that is fantastic. We might close other kinds of hospitals, but when it comes to uncovering the poor, state legislatures will be more worried than we have suggested at this conference.

Third, I think the capital markets are going to get much tighter much sooner than anybody knows. I've been waiting for the first couple of defaults of hospital bonds and I think they will come soon now that we have the DRGS.

Fourth, there has been much discussion at this conference about the necessity and desirability of closed staffs in order to get some efficiencies at the microlevel. The assumption that you can just close staffs to do that is highly questionable in my mind. As Dr. Sammons said, we'll spend the rest of the time in court. There are some management advantages if you close staffs, but I don't think that's going to be such an easy thing to do, nor do I believe it should be done unless you really think that the British or the Continental system makes a lot of sense. Nor is it a good idea to cut patients off from their conventional physician as of the moment they are hospitalized.

Fifth, we have paid practically no attention to the fact that there is not a ghost of a chance of controlling any costs, or reducing them, if we keep pushing more resources into the system, yet we're in the middle of the biggest explosion of physician manpower that we've ever seen. How are we going to control costs if each young physician who gets into the system has to make a living? Besides this explosive inflow of additional physician resources, we have a capital market with money to increase facilities, with some promise that way down the road the market will work and we will get rid of some of those excess facilities. But I see no possibility of that happening in the short run or in the midterm.

Sixth, I think it's clearly reprehensible to talk about a marketing approach to health. The notion that in the year 1984 we should really be "selling the public" on more and more stuff, a lot of which is not neutral but negative, looks to me as if the whole thing has gone berserk. What you want to do is constrain the system. You don't want to sell them more and more of what they don't need.

Seventh, as a society, we have to face up to what is the minimum acceptable level of care that is going to be available to everybody. It's quite clear that we've always had multiple levels of care. I learned that in Topeka, Kansas. In 1950 when I visited there for the first time psychiatric costs per patient were $600 a year in the Kansas Hospital, $1,800 a year at the Veterans Hospital, and $25,000 a year at the Menninger Clinic. What has to be determined, politically and socially, is the minimum acceptable care that we're going to provide for everybody by virtue of their being citizens of a semicivilized society. We haven't begun to talk about that yet because that involves the whole question of heroic interventions at the beginning and end of life and in between.

Eighth, I really believe the AMA is wrong. I think that a profession that has a leadership responsibility has to talk about its own numbers. I think I know why the AMA is so worried about talking about physician supply, but it must rethink that position. It must do something on that front, if only to tell the public that it understands the relationship between the number of physicians and the total cost to the system.

Now I want to tell you what I think will be here by 1990, which is quite different from what we're talking about. I have no reason whatever to believe that the congressional budget estimates for 1990 are wrong when they show an expenditure of $750 billion for health care, up from $362 billion in 1983. That is, I see a continuing explosive increase in the total cost of the health care system.

I think there will be a thousand things that Ford Motor Company and General Motors and General Electric and General Foods will be trying to do to get some modifications of their benefit systems, and my prophesy is that they will get very little out of all their activity.

There's no question in my mind that physicians' incomes on the average will start to slip or not go up so fast, and that there will be considerable conflicts within the physician community as to who gets positions how and with respect to what. With the increased number of physicians there will be a considerable amount of trouble and therefore I advise you not to try to do anything about closing staffs unless you want to blow the thing sky high!

I expect to see more niches. I expect for-profit medicine to find its way and pick its markets and make some dollars, and I expect some nonprofit people to do the same.

I have no reason to believe that the so-called integration approach—vertical, horizontal, or any combination thereof—is going to be any great resolution of anything. I've been impressed with the fact that the big university hospitals have had a so-called partnership. A lot of people are on the faculty. In some places, the university owns the hospital. It doesn't look like a very easy place to run.

I think the states will find great frustration. I don't think they'll be able to control very much, but they'll try. I think we'll see hospitals closing, merging, and becoming parts of larger systems, but I don't see any big cost constraints in all of this in the next six years. We'll see a lot more delivery systems, most of them probably not very good. I don't believe walk-in clinics are going to give you a very good, general level of care. You'd be better off if you walked into the emergency room of a major hospital.

I anticipate the DRG system will be manipulated by people who can manipulate it, and we will be lucky if it remains budgetarily useful.

I suspect that the system will continue to be high cost, and very mixed up with market forces, regulatory forces, for-profit forces, and nonprofit forces. I'm not at all clear how the American public will respond when we're spending $750 billion. But, at that point, we may really come to grips with the very serious political question of how a system at $750 billion will be out of control.

Let me say, as an economist interested in employment, you mustn't forget that one of the more attractive things, from politicians' points of view and from trade unions' points of view and from communities' points of view, is that health care is a very important employment sector. You put a few extra dollars in health and you offer eight million jobs for people; that's what we're offering at the present time: eight million jobs. That's two-and-a-half times the number of jobs in agriculture.

Summary II

ALAN NELSON, M.D.

I elected to view the policy implications of this great partnership from three perspectives: from the standpoint of physicians, from the standpoint of hospitals, and from the standpoint of the public.

To physicians viewing the implication of this great partnership at the crossroads, I would make four observations. First, how are physicians viewing direct competition from hospitals? How does the hospital do it? Frankly, we are being slicked from one part of the country to another. The hospital appeals to the innate allegiance or loyalty that physicians have to it. It says that the Catholic hospital down the street is setting up primary care centers and they're going to carve out their piece from our traditional catchment. We have to protect ourselves. We're already overbedded. We'd better set up some primary care centers in the neighborhood. They present that to the hospital staff and it's approved virtually without debate, certainly without any kind of major dissent.

Last week, I received in my mailbox a very nice brochure pointing out all of the advantages in terms of costs and convenience, caring and sensitivity of this practice location that has set down right smack dab in the middle of my practice in direct competition with me. The fact is, though, that I had to put up an initial investment out of my own pocket to establish my practice, and the hospital in which I practice is directly competing with me, using, either directly or indirectly, patient care dollars. That competitive center ought to give me some concern. The question is, will there be a rebellion of physicians against their hospitals for this greater competition? I honestly don't know. I certainly don't see any rebellion coming now.

The second question from the standpoint of physicians is, what is the physicians' reaction to increasing regulation coming through the hospital? I suppose one of the ways we would like to measure that is to see the reaction to the DRG system. Deep down in their souls a lot of physicians in the country think that DRG is the greatest thing since sliced bread because they see the hospitals having to confront living within a budget for the first time. The average physician is tired of being beaten about the head and shoulders about increasing costs. He wants somebody else to share some of that. He sees DRGs as one way of imposing restraints that he wanted for a long time but hasn't really known how to invoke.

In my hospital, we recently put in place a hospital formulary. It provides most medications that we need on a day-to-day basis and only a series of relatively small hurdles for us to jump over if we want drugs from the formulary. This is incredibly wise in terms of presenting us with a menu of less expensive alternative drugs and infinitely more sensible than being the victims of the detail man who is marketing the hospital pharmacy.

So, the reaction to regulation through the hospital, at least as far as DRGs are concerned, is mixed at this point. At some point, the ratcheting will reach a point where physicians will have to rebel, but that rebellion hasn't arrived.

Third, what is the physician reaction to reimbursement through the hospital? Well, we all have a great deal of fearfulness about being paid under some potential legislative process and being paid by the hospital through the DRG system. Even before we confront that, however, a lot of full-time staff physicians are sleeping very fitfully because the hospitals have more and more empty beds and the DRG system is requiring hospital administrations and medical staffs to take a look at those full-time directors of coronary care units, hospital epidemiologists, pulmonary disease specialists and others whose pay by and large comes out of patient care revenues.

Fourth, the final question from the physician perspective deals with whether competition from hospitals and the increasing physician supply requires us to aggregate. There has been a general sense in the past that physicians will have to leave solo practice and cluster into groups in order to compete more effectively and in order to market their services. I will submit that as more and more of our colleagues have empty spaces in their schedules each day, the very good physician will want to demassify, disaggregate, run lean and fast and be flexible and not carry his colleagues on his back.

Now, to discuss the policy implications of this great partnership from the standpoint of hospitals. One of the responses to the empty beds is to consolidate the catchment area with satellites and with alternative delivery settings. It is entirely possible that in doing so hospitals may lose the economies of scale they hope to achieve; that is, if they're setting up primary care centers, they have to staff those centers in a way to achieve their marketing commitments. That may not be very efficient. Such overexpansion may lead to failures. Hospitals then may find that demassification permits the leanness and flexibility they'll need to survive. There are projections that by the end of the decade all hospitals will be amalgamated into twenty large systems. I think that probably will turn out to be nonsense.

Several things will challenge hospitals. First, severe overbedding, at least partly due to public distrust of technology. When I entered practice eighteen years ago, the hospital was regarded as a haven to go to, be taken care of, get well in, and leave. Now, hospitals are regarded as a relatively dangerous place to be. I never have to talk patients out of going to the hospital anymore. In fact, I have to prove to them that they're sick enough to justify the risk.

Second, loss of what has been called the revenue center income is a big challenge for the hospital; they call it the profit center income. We will find that what used to be profit centers perhaps now will become albatrosses around their necks.

Third, we may find in some of these alternative delivery systems that the hospitals overexpand and become cost-ineffective.

What are the policy implications of this changing relationship for the public? Society, especially the purchasers of health care, want the system changed, but society has no idea what the outcome of the change it wants will be. Business thinks standard economic principles apply, but I doubt it. Business is comfortable with increasing competition, because it thinks it understands the consequences of increased competition. It thinks increased competition will decrease costs. I submit that increasing competition will inevitably increase total units of care used and total cost. It has to. Increasing competition leads to increased marketing, increased marketing leads to increased demand, increased demand leads to increased usage, and that leads to increased cost. It doesn't matter whether you knock the doctor's bill down from $22.50 to $21.00. That's not where the cost is.

The only way to decrease the rate of cost increase is to decrease facilities, decrease manpower, and decrease demand.

Throughout this conference, except for Dr. Wallace's elegant opening presentation, nobody has really talked much about cybernetics. We might apply the cybernetic model to manpower. If we're going to decrease manpower, how can we do it? Well, obviously, applying cybernetics, we have those who are promoting increased supply, nontuition funding of medical education, and the service needs of facilities, and we have three rate-limiting steps: the number of slots for students, the number of slots for residents, and the number of licenses that are granted.

Dr. Cooper told us that it doesn't look like you can very easily ration the number of slots for students. And I don't know how or if licensing bodies limit licenses. I suspect that the vulnerable place among those variables is the number of residency positions. That's where those who think the system has to be contained in terms of manpower will focus. As soon as we have many more American graduates than we have resident slots, that will have an impact on the number of slots for students as well.

Now I want to touch on four great myths that are believed by otherwise rational scholars.

The first great myth is that increased competition will contain costs. I've discussed that.

The second myth is that preventive health care will decrease costs. The better preventive health care we practice, the longer people will live; the longer people live, the more health care services they'll consume. We've said in the past that if we can find a cure for coronary artery disease, then costs will really go up. Those who now die quickly at home don't cost anybody a dime, but they'll die of something else more expensive downstream! If we are able to find a prevention for death from coronary artery disease and cancer, then the largest single expenditure for health will be nursing home care.

The third great myth that otherwise rational scholars believe is that changing the structure of the delivery system will contain costs more than just temporarily. After we've done everything we can to change the structure—we cut down on inefficiency, make all physicians work for a dollar a year, do whatever else we can do—the costs will still go up because they're a product of the number of services delivered and the number of people eligible to receive them and the technology that makes these services available.

The fourth great myth is that physicians would somehow behave the same in a system other than a fee-for-service system. We have models all over the world that show that physicians do not behave in other systems the same way they behave in the fee-for-service system. In Sweden, physicians behave in two totally different fashions on week days and weekends. On week days, they work at a very leisurely pace for the state and on weekends they work in an entirely different fashion in their home on a fee-for-service basis. This bland assumption that we can restructure the system and physicians will still continue to behave in exactly the same way is patent nonsense.

The grand alliance is at the crossroads and the key policy question is this: given that hospitals are going to be an agent to ration care after the fat and inefficiency are gone, will physicians join in the rationing or not? The answer is yes and no.

Yes, physicians will participate with society in making those global rationing decisions, defining what the benefit package is, determining where the cap on research will be placed, and deciding how many Barney Clarks will receive hearts.

No, physicians in this country will not be the rationing agent on a case-by-case basis. Here again there is a difference between our system and other modern industrialized nations. In Britain, the primary care physician is quite satisfied being the rationing point in the system. He is content to say, "Well, you know, Mum's kidneys are failing but she's getting on in years, she's sixty, so we'll make her as comfortable as we can at home." He never confronts the consultant in the hospital in making that rationing decision. I don't think that would work for a minute in this country. Primary care physicians will continue to be advocates of the patient. The big conflict between the hospital—if it is the rationing device—and the practicing physician will come when attempts are made to force the role of the rationing agent on the primary care physician on a case-by-case basis.

Discussion

PROFESSOR ENTHOVEN: First, I guess I believe in the four great myths, and I think there's quite a bit of evidence to support them.

The first thing you've got to understand is with respect to the use of terminology. When we economists talk about competition, we mean economic competition; that is, the interaction between cost-conscious buyers and cost-conscious sellers in the normal economic marketplace. The kind of competition Dr. Nelson was talking about when he said increased competition will not reduce costs is competition of providers in a cost-unconscious environment with a cost-unconscious demand side. We have a fair amount of evidence to suggest that where we make cost-conscious demands there is some reduction in cost.

Second, when you think about better preventive care reducing costs, you need to think in terms of the total social cost of illness and its treatment and not merely the expenditures on health care services. People make a terrible mistake when they confuse limiting spending with controlling costs. What Professor Reinhardt and I mean when we're talking about reducing costs is reducing the total cost of illness and its treatment.

Now, will better preventive care lead to healthier life-styles that lengthen life and reduce the burden of illness and its social cost? Yes, if you think in terms of the social cost, the burden of illness, the suffering, and the lost work time. If you understand correctly the concept of the total social cost of illness and its treatment, there is good evidence that preventive care does reduce health care costs.

Third, changing the structure of the delivery system will change costs more than just temporarily. The cost curve may go back up again, but it may go up again tracking a similar pace of growth at some 40 percent less if we have an efficient system. It also might not go up that much. Some factors like advancing technology and an aging population may cause it to go up, but it wouldn't be a bad thing if the spending went up in the context of an informed cost-conscious demand where people had choices of spending more or less.

The reason people like Professor Reinhardt and I complain about the present state of affairs is because the medical profession is able to create a cost-unconscious demand in which the de-manders of care are neither using their own money nor in any sense being financially responsible for their care, and so the present state of affairs does not respect society's preferences.

Finally, I would hope physicians would not behave the same in an alternative delivery service as in a fee-for-service system, but rather that they would behave as cost-conscious agents for their cost-conscious patients: would use resources more efficiently; would make more use of the surgicenter; would wait until technology was evaluated before they pushed it on their patients.

I have to disagree with Professor Ginzberg's comment that changing the tax laws won't work. I think we are restructuring the system successfully. A tax cap model of finance has been tried on large scale demonstrations like the multiple choice system in California. It has been tried at Stanford and Harvard universities, where there are competing HMOS, and the American Hospital Association, where Mr. McMahon tells me they offer multiple choice. To say something like this won't work merely because it is a proposed change in the tax law is a counsel of despair.

MR. BROMBERG: One, it's hard to hear Professor Ginzberg talk about eight million jobs in the health field and then say it's not a business. His proof that it's not a business is that we use the phrase "partnership" rather than "corporate health care." We have been talking about corporate health care, how physicians and hospitals are going to interrelate in a corporate health system.

Second, Professor Ginzberg made the point that the capital markets are going to turn less friendly, while Professor Enthoven commented that all the predictions about hospitals joining systems were wrong. I think Professor Ginzberg is right and Professor Enthoven is wrong. The one common denominator in for-profit and nonprofit hospitals joining systems is better access to capital, and the fear of the capital markets turning on us will just perpetuate that. I think hospitals will move together strictly for capital reasons.

Professor Enthoven's comment that competition leads to higher costs is true in some areas, but I think we have to keep in mind that the phrase "competition in health care" relates to competition among insurers, not among hospitals or physicians. You have price competition among insurers on a capitated basis so you do hold down total costs.

And, finally, if you have a tightly controlled, centrally regulated system, it is easy to predict what it will look like. But if you have a system that is more market oriented, it is almost impossible to predict because so many different things will happen. The bottom line is that the physician-hospital relationships of the future in a regulated system would be very predictable but in a market system they are going to be so varied and so multiple that it is impossible to predict what the common denominator would be.

DR. SAMMONS: Well, we finally got around to the word that I've been waiting to hear: "rationing." That is precisely what we're all talking about whether we want to admit it to ourselves or not. We are using a great many euphemisms like "prospective pricing" and "diagnosis related groupings." Yet everything that is being done is being done to ration care. The real way to reduce the total cost of health expenditures in this country is to just ration care.

Our British cousins have been doing it for many years. The Europeans are doing it in one form or another. Every system that we have looked at around the world rations care in some fashion. I have heard some of you argue that care is already rationed in this country, that it always has been on a price differential basis; that is probably true. If we're really going to talk about rationing care, then there are some things that we have to include: the impact of the hospital's increasing use of paramedical people; the increased licensure of these folks; the universities that are attempting to protect their financial base by expanding the enrollment of these sorts of people; the new role for nurses in this new system; the role of the hospital in the face of monetary restrictions and, presumably, continued reductions in admissions and length of stay and intensity of care.

I doubt seriously that there's anyone here who doesn't believe that we could live very nicely in this country, professionally and publicly, with a marked reduction in the number of medical students enrolled annually in the United States. But I suggest to you that if we're prepared to exchange the reduction in enrollments in U.S. medical schools for an increased enrollment in foreign medical shools, you'd better pay better attention to what Dr. Cooper said earlier, becaue that's exactly what will happen. Maybe the AMA does need to readdress the question of physician manpower, but I have the feeling that, if we readdress it and we say anything, we would probably say basically what I've just said. We would probably not decide to markedly reduce admissions and enrollments in the United States.

Maybe this is a good point in history to say to the Congress, "Go on and finish the job you started but didn't finish. Close the holes you created and deliberately, carefully, and methodically left open."

The spread of technology, however expensive it is, carries with it some overwhelming, irrefutable reasons for its continued development and dissemination. The one thing that gets missed in all of this is the quality of life. I wouldn't argue for two minutes that doing a coronary bypass is going to extend anyone's life expectancy by very much, if at all, but having been one of those people who has had a coronary, I would rather have a coronary bypass than to have another coronary because of the quality of life differential.

Let me just ask a question. In the light of everything that you know about the system and the American people and their abilities and their wants and their desires, what are you going to spend health care dollars for when you quit spending them on health? Those eight million people employed in health care are the same kinds of people who buy new automobiles, buy life insurance, send their kids to Duke, pay their school taxes, and buy food, clothing, and groceries.

What is the ultimate reason for attempting to change the system? Is this an exercise that we're going through because somebody doesn't have anything else to do? Or is there some real good, valid reason for saying that spending on health care of the American people is too great a percentage of the gross national product? If there is a real valid reason for that, then what is it? What are you going to spend it for when you quit spending it on health care for the American people?

I think that at some point we ought to have a carefully put together seminar and look at the impact of the increasing number of paramedicals involved in the system at a time when the system is under attack for unnecessary or inefficient expenditures. We'd better start looking at the impact of the paramedical people on the total cost of care and what the educational institutions are doing to protect their turf and their income by expanding those kinds of acitivities in the university setting.

PROFESSOR GINZBERG: It is a serious misinterpretation to assume that the physicians have been driving this system in its very high cost expansion. That happened very simply when we moved to Medicare and Medicaid and put that on top of the prepayment system we had earlier. When we moved to 90 percent hospital reimbursement from third parties we simply took all dollar controls off the system. To say that the physicians have been driving that system is ridiculous.

What really happened was that the federal government made a commitment to bring in the poor and the elderly. They gave them access to the hospitals without understanding that if they were just going to pay all the bills, the bills were going to get very large. I would argue that what really got the present system out of gear was a lack of understanding of the implications of moving to a 70 percent prepayment through the whole of the system. We had an economically restrained medical system in the old days because no hospital could spend more than its voluntary trustees were able to come up with, period. In 1965 we made a pipeline to the U.S. Treasury, and we have taken a very long time to adjust to that.

It makes some sense to worry about why the system shouldn't continue to go indefinitely the way it has been going. The amount of pressure now on the federal budget and, more importantly, on state budgets, is really squeezing other important systems. You just can't walk away and say it is of no significance. I would like to see more money put into education rather than just indefinitely on the health front.

My main point is that I don't think the doctors did anything but respond to the environment. Society, not the doctors, said the dollars don't count anymore.

MR. MCNERNEY: Up until recently, we've pretty well convinced ourselves that the states were not going to play a particularly prominent role because they lack money, too; many of them were broke; and they lack the administrative machinery to be very effective. Do I hear you saying that that is going to change significantly? Do you predict at the same time that the federal government will continue to play a rather recessive role?

Three years ago we were convinced that capital was going to be very tight, and yet the hospitals have done quite well in competing with railroads, with educational institutions, and with everybody. I just don't see the evidence yet that that's happening.

I'm not sure that hospitals will restrict medical staffs at risk, particularly with growing numbers of doctors. Why are they going to be at risk, particularly as economics drives this system toward more price sensitivity?

Finally, is there some evidence that preventive services and health promotion in fact reduce absenteeism or have a salubrious impact on drug abuse or smoking? Do they improve productivity at work, reduce accidents, and affect other things that are very important to the employer?

PROFESSOR ENTHOVEN: I was thinking of studies of Breslow and others that show that healthy life-styles lead to better health.

DR. ELLWOOD: I don't think it's an issue of whether or not preventive programs work. If they did, wouldn't they be a good idea to do? That's like saying, let's not give people polio vaccine because they will just live longer!

DR. OTTENSMEYER: The concept that the greatest virtue that drives the medical profession is the fee-for-service, office-based, independent practice of medicine, and that anybody who does otherwise is lazy, slothful, and unproductive is utter nonsense. Beyond that, it is an unfortunate implication that has been a party line in the establishment of medicine for thirty years. I think saying that the fee-for-service system is the only virtue that drives the medical profession is a real indictment of the ethics of the profession as well as a poor system of motivation. I think the profession and the American Medical Association should be looking very hard at the entrenched concepts that we have of medicine, such as the fee-for-service system. We must look at alternatives if we're going to take part in the changes that are so obviously necessary.

PROFESSOR DANZON: I would like to suggest the economic framework for looking at the question of organization, cost control, quality control, and the policy implications. In Economics I, many of you learned that there are two conditions of economic efficiency: one is efficiency in production in which you produce a particular type of service at the minimum cost; the other is what is called an "occasional efficiency" and that means you're allocating resources efficiently to different uses. Essentially, that means that the marginal return per dollar spent is the same for different uses.

The obvious challenge to this notion in health care is that we cannot measure benefits, but the fact is that when you make choices—which we have to do when we have budget constraints—you are implicitly evaluating benefits, so we might as well try and do it explicitly.

Given those two notions of efficiency, the public policy questions—to an economist looking at alternative forms of organization or reimbursement—are, which forms of organization will lead to more efficient allocation of resources if rationing is done by physicians or by hospitals or by insurance companies or by businesses? And which services will be covered and which ones won't?

We have to accept the fact that there will be limits on the health care budget. I would like to suggest that different organizational forms should be chosen by their efficiency and rationing.

I don't accept the notion that an increase in the supply of physicians or paraprofessionals has or will necessarily increase health care costs. Over the last two decades there have been government programs; there has been a tremendous increase in subsidies to the private sector through tax deductibility; there has been growth in other forms of financing hospitals; there has been aging of the population and growth of income. All of those things—not just the increasing number of physicians—have driven up expenditures on health care.

MR. SHELTON: I agree with Professor Ginzberg's forecast of $750 billion health care expenditures by 1990, given business as usual. That's one of the reasons why employers like Ford Motor Company are very concerned about what's happening in health care costs. For many years we watched our costs double every five years.

The level of concern has escalated to a point where I think some dramatic actions will be taken in the next year or so. I think those actions are going to be supported by labor, because business and labor both recognize that the present benefit structure with its improper incentives contributes to the costs and, more importantly, that the reimbursement in place, namely fee-for-service, is largely responsible for what has happened to costs.

What is business going to do? Four things will happen.

One, there is going to be an intense effort to try to change the benefit package. Where management can do that unilaterally, they will. For example, we put in a copayment deductible for our salaried people in January of this year and we were able to do it because we didn't have to negotiate with the union. At the same time, we offered them comprehensive coverage through a series of HMOs. We will continue to expand those alternatives so that they have choices other than the traditional Blue Cross and Blue Shield fee-for-service program. Interestingly, the salaried people flocked to this program.

Two, large employers are developing data systems that will enable them to identify providers of services who are out of line either on a cost or a utilization basis. We are putting in place a program with Med-Stat that will allow us to develop profiles on providers. The intent is that these data systems will allow us, working with labor, to develop what I call limited access, capitated programs.

Three, the business community is moving toward those limited access, capitated programs that draw upon paramedical services to a greater extent than any programs we have at present.

Four, the business community, through its frustrations, is going to continue to support regulation. In the state of Michigan, for example, we are introducing a hospital capital expenditure limitation program. There is a labor-business coalition that is going to lobby very hard to see that through. There will also be legislation that limits reimbursement of providers. In Michigan we also have a hospital capacity reduction program, the only one to my knowledge in the country. It calls for a 3,800 bed reduction in the state over a five year period, 2,500 in the city of Detroit. As you might expect, we have had intense lobbying from the providers involved. These are the kinds of things that the business community, out of its frustration, is going to be doing.

The business community is working very aggressively to bring its costs in line. We would like to be able to price our products so that the hospital workers will go out and buy two Fords rather than one. Health care costs represent the largest component in our wage and benefit package other than the wage itself and the cost-of-living provision. We did a comparison of our health care costs with the Japanese and we found that our costs were six times higher than their costs, including the government's share of the cost.

Much of what I have heard at this conference was about how we can protect our market share, how we as doctors or as hospitals can take care of our particular needs. I didn't hear much conversation about what are we going to do about unnecessary utilization. What are we going to do about unit costs that are out of line? What are we going to do with all this excess capacity? We just seem to accept it and say, well, maybe it's all right and rather than health care costs equalling 10 percent of GNP, maybe they ought to take 20 percent and everybody will be happy. I submit to you that the business community and labor are not going to be happy. They're going to be taking some very dramatic actions. They may be the wrong things, so we need the support of the provider community to help us do the right things.

DR. COOPER: One can look at how big our medical school classes are from two points of view. The one that is typical for all other education is to provide opportunity for all students who are qualified and interested in studying medicine. As a matter of fact, in 1968 the AMA and the AAMC said that every individual in this country who is qualified and who is interested in studying medicine should be provided an opportunity to do so.

The second way is to say that we're going to produce only the number of physicians that somebody thinks the country needs. I don't know who the "somebody" is who is going to tell us how many we need.

Why is it that people are worried about physicians? The reason is that 70 percent of the cost of health care is prepaid. There is no other business like it, and people are jealous of that kind of business. They don't want that kind of business to continue.

Suppose somebody tells us how many physicians we need, how are we going to control them? In 1984 we have been attempting to get 7,900 U.S.-born and foreign graduates of foreign medical schools into an approved residency program. We're graduating about 16,500 in addition. You can see that the number trying to come into this country from outside is really very large in comparison with what we ourselves are producing. How can we keep those people out? We could expand the requirement that ten states have, that a physician cannot legally practice medicine without at least one year—or maybe two or three years—of residency training. Residency training will be the final common pathway for physicians educated abroad or in this country. We could probably control it better through this pathway, but there are political implications here. The American graduates of foreign medical schools are developing a political base in the states and from time to time in the federal government.

Since we finished the health care system, I'd like to look at the automobile manufacturing system.

The question is, should we limit the number of cars produced by our automobile manufacturers? Cars have a social price. The more cars they produce, the more roads we have to build, and that comes out of tax dollars. Cars add to our balance of payments deficits. We import oil; a lot of it goes to automobiles, and it also goes into petrochemicals which are used in producing tires. Cars produce pollution which requires tax money.

The more automobiles we produce, the worse it is for the health of our public. They produce accidents; one of the biggest causes of death in those below the age of thirty is automobiles. They destroy all these young lives and raise the cost of health care which somebody has to pay for. They require us to hire more police to go out and maintain the speed limits and all the other things on the highway. Now we have the problem of imports. We have tried putting a voluntary limit on the number of cars that come in.

In the USSR, they have very few cars and very few roads, a much simpler system. Maybe we ought to put a limit on the number of cars that can be produced in this country because of the social cost of those cars.

We can look at a lot of systems that have some of the same problems that we've been addressing with medicine.

DR. BOYLE: A number of questions have been addressed that I find of extraordinary importance. When economists decide they are going to provide the prescription for restructuring the system, they ought to have in mind the possibility that there may be social consequences different from those economic models.

Physicians are engaged in a life role, to which they dedicated themselves perhaps in undergraduate school, which is taking care of patients. That is what the whole system was all about. We seem to be drifting away from that objective. Now we are addressing our attention much more seriously to how do we get a share of the market, how do we become involved in partnerships? What we ought to be talking about is how we can rededicate ourselves as a profession in a social milieu in which we have to become much more involved in making economic decisions. Are we willing to listen to economists when they come to us? Are we willing to listen when Professor Reinhardt talks about costs and quality? If we're going to approach this, we all need help.

MR. MCMAHON: I continue to wonder why we have so much difficulty addressing the topic. I guess it's because one never can reach a conclusion if there are differences in assumptions. I addressed myself earlier—clearly without persuading anybody or even achieving understanding—to the fact that there seem to be differences between those who would like to achieve social and economic ends with greater marketplace incentives and those who think that regulation is the better way to do it. Professor Ginzberg sees a very definite trend toward state regulation, and I think that's tragic.

I see another bar to moving toward some conclusions and that is the issue of what a change in the rate of increase of health care expenditures does. Some people are still absolutely persuaded that a decrease in the rate of increase from 15 or 16 percent down to 10, 9, or 8 percent is going to lead to a reduction in quality and to rationing. Others of us think appropriate changes can eliminate unnecessary expenditures.

When we put into place those three marvelous spending engines—Blue Cross and Blue Shield, Medicare, and Medicaid—we provided tremendous incentives to expand the system, and so we did it. Hospitals did it. Physicians did it. Statistics now show reductions in admissions, reductions in lengths of stay, and reductions in testing. We have come down markedly from a 15 percent rate of increase on the hospital side to 9 percent.

DR. ROGERS: The only way that Wilbur Cohen was able to get Medicare and Medicaid passed was through doctors, through that provision that there was going to be "business as usual" in the health care system. I don't think that's something the medical profession should feel very proud of. We're partly to blame for this. Yet that program did exactly what it was intended to do and it did it very well. That's a remarkable American achievement. It brought virtually all of our indigent into the health care system; it brought the poor, and it brought the blacks. We have some very striking improvements in health statistics. I don't think we should criticize it as much as we have. It was an elegant social program. I agree that there are other social priorities now in a time of economic decline and we've got to be more responsible.

You ask about quality. The public doesn't care about that. They say it's costing too much. If we remain insensitive to that, we do it at great peril.

I do not think it necessarily follows that if we magically dissolve all the sludge in people's arteries, if we don't have any more coronary artery disease, and if we cure cancer that we will inevitably end up with more costs. It is conceivable that, if we can develop a society in which we all live out our four score and ten, the costs will increase, but that period of infirmity at the end is not being extended infinitely. I don't like the discouragement in that notion. It is highly probable that we will continue to nibble away at those very big killers with the hope we all won't end up in nursing homes as an inevitable accompaniment to the end of life.

MR. ROGERS: I agree with Mr. Shelton that the impact of industry on the health care field may be as great as the impact of government action. I see Lee Iacocca, for instance, calling for the government not only to bail out Chrysler as a corporation, but now to help in his health care problem by calling for national health insurance.

For years, Congress has been talking about doing something about cost containment. That judgment has now been made in an administration which came to power saying it was going to deregulate. The medical profession had better watch it carefully because I expect DRGs will be expanded to bring in doctors. The threshold has been crossed, and government will play a more and more active role in setting some cost restraints.

Overall, I think the health industry is going to adjust itself pretty well. There will be changes. The large hospitals may be overbedded for a while, but maybe they'll use those beds for something else. They'll be moving into nursing care or whatever. I think they're going to do more and more home health care. This is an inevitable movement, and it will be coordinated more and more with the central hospital. We're seeing it already with some major institutions. They're doing the planning now to be able to go out and deliver health care to the whole area. This will be the movement and, of course, costs will always be a major concern.

PROFESSOR REINHARDT: I want to come back once more to the issue of the physician supply. In 1972, some of us started to see a surplus and began to worry about health manpower. We belonged to the Parkinsonian school which believed that physicians could just induce demand and that would increase health care expenditures.

In retrospect I think I may have been wrong. It is indeed true that, as the physician supply has increased, expenditures on physicians' services have increased pretty much proportionately. The number of visits per capita hasn't increased. Visits per physician have gone down. But billing per visit has gone up, not just price—it's more intensive services. It's possible that by having more physicians, more innovative things can be done on the delivery side because there are enough doctors. So, it may not be right to look just at physicians' billings as an index of what's happening to health care. We must also not forget that it is, in fact, a constitutional issue to artificially restrict entry into a way of life.

PROFESSOR STEVENS: We have been critical of physicians. We have talked about the very large number of physicians coming into medical practice in this decade and the next decade. We have heard about anxiety; the role of physicians in stimulating accessible change at the local level; and the need of physicians to deal with organizations of one sort or another. But we have skirted the whole issue of how far physicians are going to maintain or abrogate their traditional responsibility for designing and articulating patient care. We keep avoiding this as though physicians will be irrelevant in decision making in the next decade.

Then there's the question of the role of the profession in this business-oriented enterprise that we've been talking about. I think that increasingly over the next few years we're going to come back to the role of the physician as the decision maker, and what it means to be a member of the profession in the late twentieth century.

DR. DUVAL: All I'll do is observe the old saw that where one stands depends upon where one sits. I was impressed at how easy it was for many of us to make observations about the shortcomings of physicians and hospitals and systems and insurers and payers and government, business, and industry, in short, whatever segment the speaker was not a part of.

DR. EUGENE STEAD: You know, the one thing we've left out of this whole business is science. Since World War II we've made tremendous investigations and discoveries about how biological systems work. Once we got over the antibiotic era, scientific discoveries paid off relatively little at the health care level. But they are going to pay off tremendously in the future. We tend to talk here as if the health care phase is going to be what we decide today. But there's going to be a tremendous revolution in what medical care is as medical practice begins to put the output of the past thirty years of science actually to work.

PROFESSOR GINZBERG: I don't think the federal government is going to tackle the tax issue. I also don't think it's going to tackle the physician issue until you take some leadership. We may have a chance of getting Congress to close some loopholes, if you really stand up and make lots of noise, but until you start to make noise nothing is going to happen.

The Congress must act on Medicare and the trust funds and they'd better not try to cut the benefits; they'd better try to get the revenues up.

Since the federal government can't really lean effectively on the different localities of this country, the nearest instrument that you have is state legislatures. They may do it very poorly but they're under different pressures which I think will get them to move. One of these days they may even come in through the back door on the medical education front. I would expect local practitioners in the states to lean against the legislatures and say, "What are you doing taking our tax money to create more competition for us? Why don't you reduce medical school classes a bit?"

I don't know much about capital markets, but I would suspect with the interest rates going up and with Congress looking at the industrial bond tax-free affair with a dubious eye that all we need are a couple of defaults on payments—which are going to come under DRGs—and that will change the market for hospital loans.

On the matter of medical staff closure, I think those staffs that are closed now can stay closed and I expect a few more to be able to close, but I raise the issue of who the hospital belongs to. Most community hospitals belong in some loose way to the community which will make it extremely difficult, in my perception, to close them. Nor do I believe they should be closed for so-called economic efficiency if there is a considerable social disutility. I don't like to see more and more physicians close down hospitals. That's not my idea of how the system gets better. I'm perfectly willing to see standards set and used reasonably as to who can come in, but I don't want to close physicians out arbitrarily.

What Mr. Shelton reported offering Ford employees who are salaried is going on and it will accelerate. But the issue here is whether that will be cost reducing or cost shifting. My own hunch is that it includes a little bit of cost reduction but most of it will be cost shifting. Even the amount of cost shifting that you will be able to do with your employees is pretty limited.

I wrote my first piece in 1959 in *The New England Journal of Medicine*, and I said, "You're going to buy yourselves all kinds of troubles by pushing too many physicians in." But I don't think the doctors will be at the wrong end of the stick in the end. I think we will shift dollars. We now have a 40/20 split in the dollars between the hospitals and doctors. If you can get six or seven percentage points off the hospital, you can take care of the physicians, and that's what I think lies in the background of a lot of this push toward ambulatory care.

I had some experience running the biggest health system that was ever run in the United States on efficiency terms. I controlled all the doctors, all the nurses, and everybody else in the U.S. medical system in World War II. I was the chief logistical advisor to the Surgeon-General of the Army. And I learned that the only resource I wanted to control was the manpower going in because that was the scarce resource.

I'm a political economist and I cannot leave out of the equation the cost of social transformation. I will not vote for taking the inequalities out of tax deductions on insurance unless I do it on oil exploration and a lot of other depreciation accounts. What we are now facing is a tremendously difficult way to find the social levers to affect any part of this system. The system is going to run from seven or eight contradictory places. The states are going to make a mess out of it, but they're going to be in it. There's no question that the market is going to have some influence. There are doctors coming in that you'd like to control, but you don't know how. You're going to shift some costs, but you're not going to reduce the total costs very much, and that's the nature of the business. There's no escape from that particular beast until you get into a very much worse position than we're in now, because we're not in that bad a position.

We can go from 11 percent of the GNP spent on health care to somewhere around 15 percent and maybe then you'll get a real set of political pressures from the public to do something, but not now.

DR. NELSON: I was asked whether the trend of physicians to get into groups might turn itself around, and I freely admit I have no data. I draw some inferences from my own observations, but the observations are based on the understanding that six or eight or ten physicians in a group share the overhead. It's very difficult to cut the overhead as the volume of patients decreases, because we can't engage in flexible staffing. So, they have the same overhead and fewer patients and, as soon as some of those physicians have large parts of their days unfilled and can't produce anything, the high producers are trapped and want to offload.

I also sense that new physicians entering practice are not as comfortable with the security traditionally sought in group practices because they don't know if that bigger group will be flexible enough. If they are entrepreneurial at all, they're more willing to take the risk that comes with capital expenditure and referral patterns.

Dr. Ottensmeyer implied that I was reflecting the old traditional AMA party line, favoring fee-for-service as opposed to structured practice settings. At this conference we speak as individuals. We have plenty of people representing structured, non-fee-for-service models at this meeting, and I happen to be reflecting my own bias on the type of system that I happen to have chosen, in presenting some of the counterbalancing arguments. I would add, though, that AMA data do clearly show that physicians practicing in a structured setting work fewer hours a week than do fee-for-service physicians.

I doubt that we will get into rationing until the fat has been cut in the benefit package. The benefit package has to be altered for patients who would benefit from a particular service and are not able to receive that service because of cost only. I don't know when or if that will come, but I happen to think that at some point we're going to have to put a cutoff at sixty years old for a renal transplant, and eighty years old for a coronary artery procedure, for instance. When that comes, when patients can't have what they can't pay for, that's rationing!

Finally, let me clearly state my own personal support for all preventive medical activities. It's the best investment we can make. It's an investment in the quality of care, in the quality of life, and in the productivity of our citizenry. In my view, it is not necessarily an investment that will pay off in terms of decreased health care costs. But that shouldn't matter. It's like my advice to my patients about jogging; I'm not sure it will prevent them from having a coronary, but if they feel better afterward it's like virtue having its own reward. Obviously we are all in favor of preventive medicine as an important contribution to health.

Index